MASSAGE THERAPY

The principles and practice of holistic massage which treats the body as a complex balance of mental, physical and spiritual aspects, bringing health and harmony to mind and body.

MASSAGE THERAPY

The holistic way to physical and mental health

by

Richard Jackson

Photographs by Selby Smith
Illustrations by Bonnie Timmons

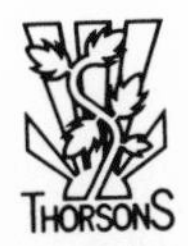

THORSONS PUBLISHERS LIMITED
Wellingborough, Northamptonshire

First published in the United Kingdom 1980
*Original American edition published by
Drake Publishers Inc., New York*

ISBN 0 7225 0646 5

Printed and bound in Great Britain by
Biddles Ltd., Guildford, Surrey.

Contents

Illustrations

Preface

Holistic Massage is composed of three parts—*The Mind, The Body,* and *The Spirit.* This is in accordance with the holistic philosophy, which views health as a balance of these three aspects of life.

Part I: "The Mind: Aspects of Holistic Massage." When friends inquire about this book, I tell them that it is a health book in a massage format. The many concepts related to holistic health found within these pages can be used in any health practice. I have tried to show how these concepts can be applied to massage. I leave it to the reader to find ways to integrate the holistic philosophy into all levels of health and daily living. Holistic thought can be applied to much more than massage, and I hope this material will stimulate you to do just that.

The difference between holistic massage and conventional massage is that the former integrates newer ideas of holistic health with long established techniques of massage. Massage does not need to be considered simply as a mechanical art. When more elements are added to the basic massage technique, it turns out to be a dynamic health process.

So Part I is a basic introduction to some of the concepts of holistic health and how they relate to holistic massage. In it are contained many *experiences* in self-awareness that reinforce the text material. I encourage you to try these exercises if you sincerely wish to experience holistic massage and not just to understand it intellectually. Reading books is usually a merely mind-oriented matter, and the exercises suggested throughout this book are meant to help you avoid that.

The holistic philosophy of health has not as yet been formalized; its youth renders it quite nebulous. But a foundation, an order to many scattered thoughts, is now beginning to emerge. The concepts presented in Part I are by no means a complete exposition of holistic thought. Rather, I have presented some ideas and practices relating to the physical body that are relevant to an understanding of holistic massage.

Holistic thought so far has not been practically applied to everyday health practices. It has emerged through a series of excellent books that examine and evaluate our present health-care system. A new view of health and sickness, and the health-care system, seems to be in order, but there have not been extensive writings on *how* these ideas can be applied. I have tried to bring the holistic theory and ideas presented in Part I down to a practical, experiential level.

Part II: "The Body: Massage Technique." If you are simply interested in learning how to give a conventional massage, then turn to this section without further delay. Here you will find the actual mechanics of massage reduced to the essence. Everything you need to know to give an excellent massage is explained within a few short pages.

Massage technique is relatively easy to grasp. There are only a few mechanical movement patterns to master. Massage books in the past have burdened the learner with long elaborations on various strokes. I feel that this tends to hinder rather than help. It is important to grasp the basic, logical structure of massage and then allow the varieties of strokes to develop on their own. Expertise naturally follows with experience.

This section does give a structural outline for holistic massage, but for the actual techniques of focusing (an integral part of holistic massage), the reader will have to continue on and read the third section, "The Spirit."

Part III: "The Spirit: Holistic Massage Experiences." This section was particularly difficult to write. Michael, a close friend who wrote the last chapter, "The Receiver," also had a trying time with this part. Words fail when one tries to express spiritual concepts and feelings. After all, what is the meaning of spiritual? Each of us has his own feelings and definitions of this aspect of his life. It is very likely that one person's experience is never exactly like another's. Too, the spiritual experiences of giver and receiver depend directly on set, setting, and circumstance. Their personal backgrounds and inclinations play a large role. The important point is to realize that the spiritual aspect of oneself *can* play a significant role in the total massage experience. Whether one chooses to travel these roads or not depends upon the individual, but the roads do exist for those so inclined.

I have included a preliminary chapter in Part III, "Meditation and Focusing." This material, combined with the first two parts of the book, will enable the reader to realize some of the mental and spiritual possibilities of holistic massage. The last two chapters, "The Giver" and "The Receiver," do not completely describe the experiences possible for massage partners by any means. They only give clues and representative examples that can show the reader some of the possibilities of holistic massage. These chapters should be used as an informational guide and not combed for specific goals to strive for.

The best advice I have to offer is for you to view this book as a whole. Read it in its entirety before attempting to understand holistic massage. Try to practice the many experiences found throughout these pages. Allow the holistic approach to massage to develop and grow as you change and grow through practice. There are many concepts to examine, and it is up to you, the reader, to integrate these ideas into the massage experience. Holistic health and massage are not cure-alls; they are not panaceas for all our ills. Rather, they suggest a new way of perceiving health, of seeing our condition from another perspective.

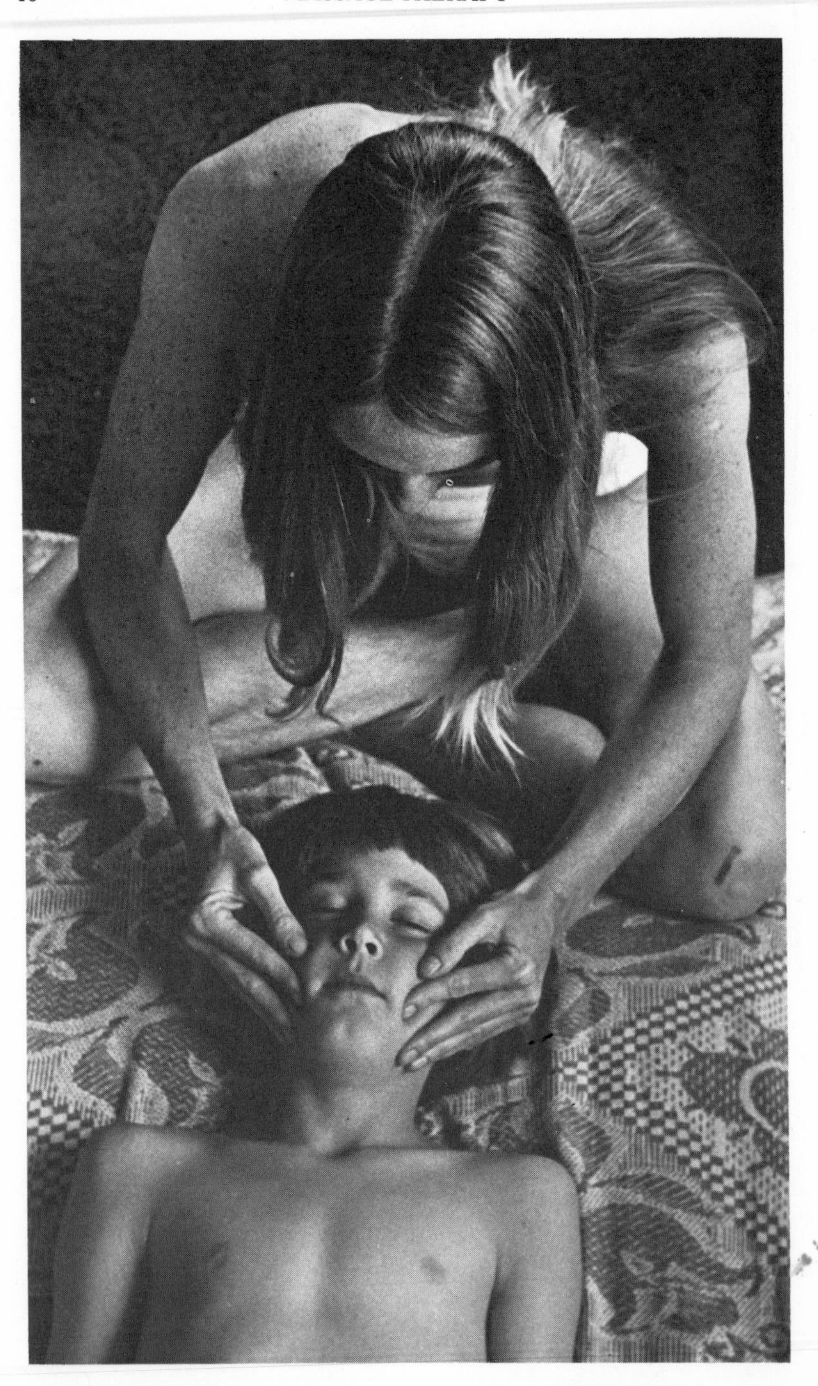

"I get by with a little help from my friends."

Acknowledgements

A number of people helped in the creation of this book. First, I owe a debt of gratitude to Selby Smith. Had it not been for him, I never would have started this project. He not only encouraged me to write my ideas down, he also guided me during the long months of writing by criticizing my work and making endless suggestions. His constant prodding and encouragement was a primary factor in the completion of *Holistic Massage*. The photography found throughout these pages is also Selby's work. I sincerely thank him for seeing the project through to the end.

Another friend, Michael Flavin, also deserves recognition and my sincerest thanks. Michael spent weeks editing the manuscript and offering advice, and it was he who wrote the last chapter, "The Receiver." If I ever learn to construct a proper sentence, I will have Michael to thank for it.

I thank Bill Paff for helping me see the ways in which massage can be more than a mechanical experience. His sensitivity and knowledge contributed to the birth of holistic massage.

Thanks also to Bonnie Timmons, who is responsible for the graphics. There were many long days of work, especially as the deadline approached. She was a constant source of ideas, and her feedback helped immeasurably during the final rewrite of the manuscript. Thanks also to Dennis Forbis for his help with the graphics.

In addition to the people I have mentioned, I also want to thank Holly, Tom, Kathy, Lisette, Peggy, Richard, and Kris for reading the manuscript and offering constructive criticisms.

A special thanks goes to my wife, Kathy, for the long hours she has spent typing, typing, and retyping again. She has always encouraged me to write, and when I started, she never questioned what I was doing. This was the greatest help of all.

PART 1

THE MIND: ASPECTS OF HOLISTIC MASSAGE

"It is a mistake to think the only way to help a sick man is to take away his illness . . ."

—Rolling Thunder

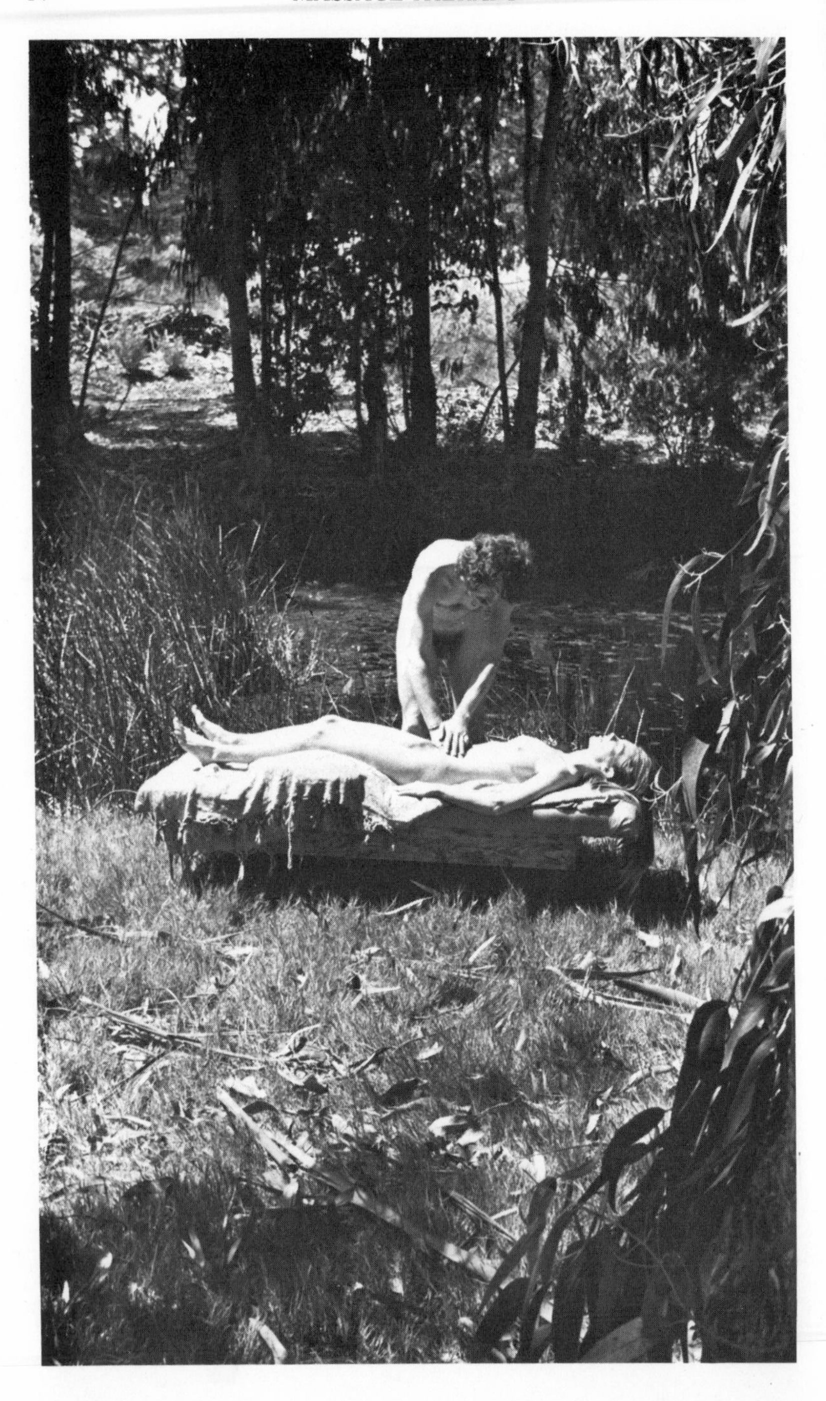

1.

Holistic Health and Massage

Health care is changing. Today we are witnessing a revisioning of attitudes toward health care that is taking us back in time to a more personalized form of health care and ahead toward new ways of viewing health and healing. The term that describes this new health is "holistic," from the Greek *holos*, meaning "whole." It is based on the belief that an organic or integrated whole has a reality independent of and greater than the sum of its parts. The greater reality of any whole, including holistic health and massage, cannot be fully understood until there exists an awareness and understanding of the many aspects, or component parts, that comprise the whole. I think these aspects are best understood by contrasting holistic health philosophy with present-day medical practice.

The first aspect to consider is the holistic definition of health. Health is not seen as simply the absence of illness. It is a dynamic process—*not* a static state. There are degrees of health, and it is up to the individual to determine how close he or she will come to optimal health. Today we have a tendency to isolate an illness and dwell on it, saying that we are sick, instead of viewing our whole condition and seeing that the total balance is overwhelmingly on the side of health.

The holistic practitioner views sickness in relation to the organism as a whole. Health is considered a balance of the physical, mental, and spiritual aspects of life. If this balance is upset, sickness results. The individual is viewed as the *only* person capable of maintaining that balance. The cause of most illness is to be found within the individual and in his relationship to the environment and to other people. Treatment of symptoms is not enough. Eliminating the cause of illness is more important, and this can be done only by the individual. Disease may be triggered by an external force, such as a germ or a virus, but the cause is ultimately seen as originating from within the individual. We need to change the assumption that we are at the mercy of indiscriminate attack by disease or disease-causing organisms. This assumption strips us of any responsibility for our own health. The public feels that it has little or no control over its health and healing. The cause of illness is laid at the feet of chance, and the cure is the exclusive property of the physician. The individual is transformed into an anesthetized bystander. The Western medical model is self-propagating because it systematically strips people of their natural abilities to heal themselves. Studies have shown that the greatest determinants of good health are personal health habits governing eating, smoking, drinking, and so on; environmental factors; and, most important, thoughts and attitudes. These factors are under the control of the individual, *not* the medical community. The individual must make positive changes affecting health before positive health can be reached.

The holistic health philosophy considers the body as a dynamic energy system which is in a constant state of change. Human beings are more than just their bodies. Each is a complex balance of mental, physical, and spiritual aspects that are integrated into, and affected directly by, environmental and social factors. The gestalt of mind/body/spirit cannot be fragmented or isolated, and the cause of an illness is more important than external symptoms. This attitude is the polar opposite of current medical theory and practice, which fragments the body. We live in an age of specialization in which medical specialization is but one manifestation of the larger tendency toward scientific specialization. Each part of the body is viewed and treated as separate from the rest of the body. Researchers take great pains to isolate that which they are studying, and they try to eliminate all other variables. Experiments are carried out with a sterility and detachment that prevents the results from being useful in everyday life. In addition to fragmenting the physical body, our "modern" approach is to fragment the human unit into its physical, mental, and spiritual aspects as well. It is not unusual today to see the body fragmented in research and treatment, rather than integrated and viewed as a whole. Research studies that take into account emotional and environmental

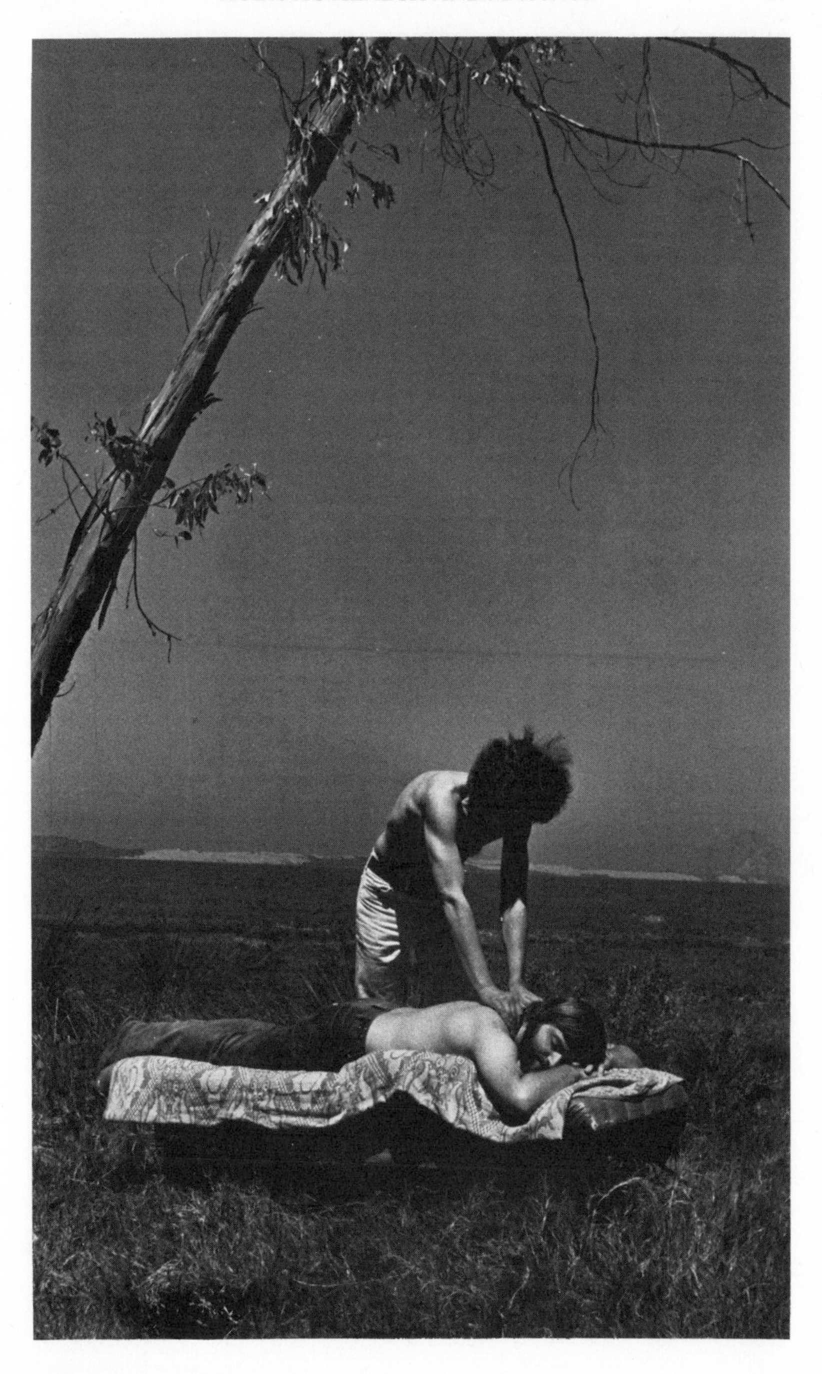

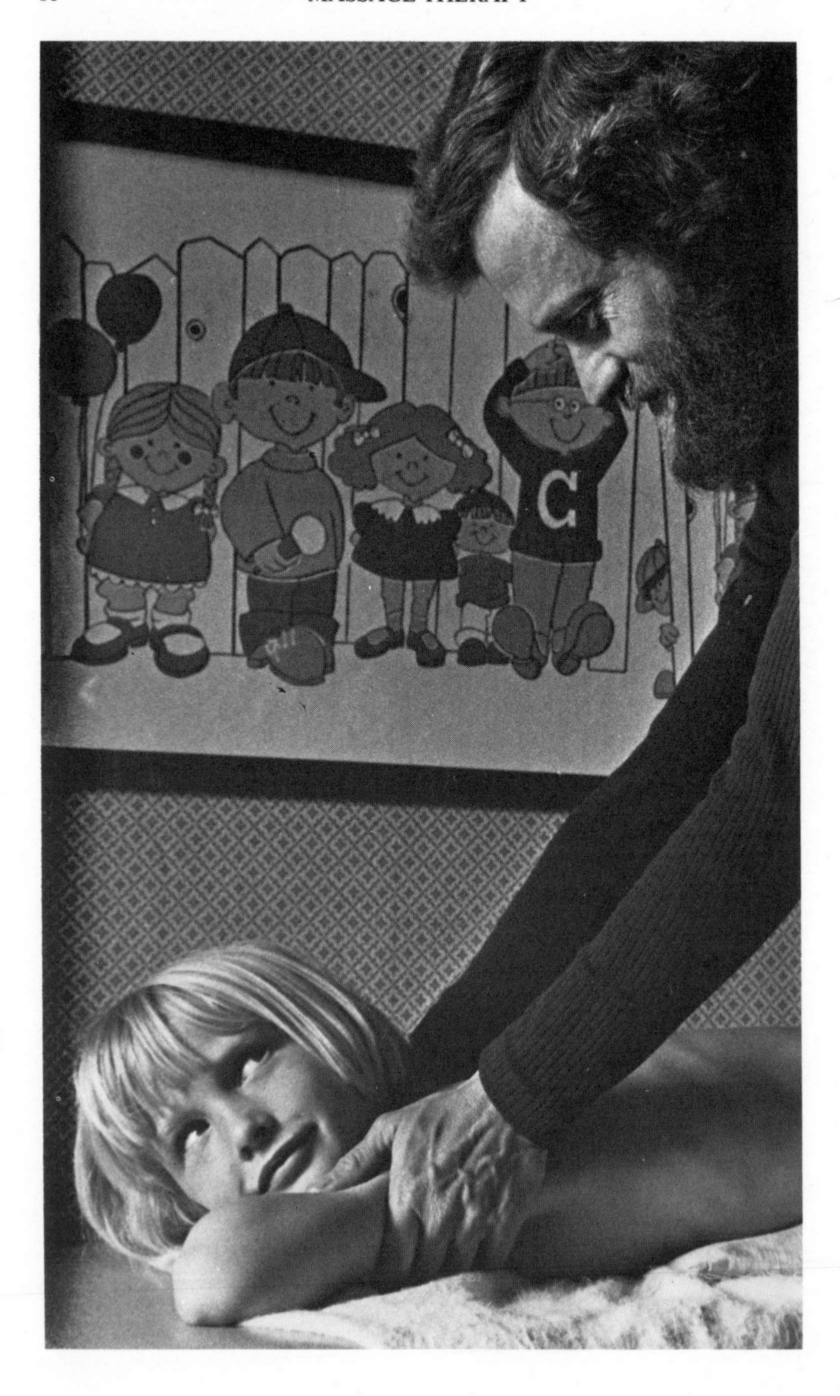

variables, as well as subjective data, are frowned upon as invalid.

Western medicine has explored and technologically refined three areas of healing: diagnosis, medicines/chemotherapy, and surgery. Medical science has virtually ignored other important approaches to sickness and health. It has done comparatively little to improve the over-all health of the population and to find the true *causes* of illness, so that they can be dealt with effectively. The explanation we have been given for the cause of disease is termed the "germ theory," because it indicates that disease is caused by microorganisms that attack us without cause or provocation and make us ill. This does not mean that doctors think *all* disease or illness is caused by germs. If illness is not attributed to invasion of the body by microorganisms, then diseases such as cancer, heart disease, and multiple sclerosis are often labeled "cause unknown." This prevalence of the "cause unknown" designation has persisted throughout the years because medical science is most concerned with the *effects*, or symptoms, of illness, rather than the *causes*. Treating the symptoms is the general rule. Modern medicine has neglected to examine or treat the causes of illness adequately, a neglect due mainly to unsound root assumptions about the body. Until they change their basic ideas about the structure and functioning of the organism as a balanced whole in relation to its environment, the "modern" medical professionals will make little progress in understanding the disease process. The rules of scientific methodology and investigation must also be restructured to include important variables which have been previously ignored.

The holistic approach to treatment rests in searching for the cause of the "dis-ease" within the individual or in his relation to his environment and then eliminating the cause. Education plays an important role in this type of treatment. The patient is responsible for his or her health, or the lack of it, and it is the responsibility of the health worker to give the patient the knowledge and tools he needs to effect positive health changes within himself. Holistic health workers are used as resources for good health. Their method of treatment takes a great deal of time, but the results are often more effective and longer-lasting than our present form of symptomatic care. Unfortunately, many of the drugs employed for symptomatic treatment tend to shut down the body's normal defense mechanisms. The body loses the capacity to care for itself, subsequently relying on more drugs to make it well. Many drugs have side effects which may be more severe than the illness for which they are prescribed. Our society has an incredible reliance on drugs. The fact is that most drugs do not *cure* anything. Rather, they only mask the patient's symptoms and make the sickness more tolerable.

The area of major emphasis in holistic health is hardly considered in present medical practice. The holistic practitioner is concerned primarily with prevention of disease. This entails much more than an annual physical. Prevention includes the education and individual responsibility I have already discussed. Active prevention and health maintenance is truly *health* care, methods which contrast considerably with our present system of sick care.

The aspects of Western medicine I have described add up to a situation in which the individual becomes dependent on doctors and drugs to maintain health. The individual is not seen as creating his own illness or health. Therefore, little effort is made to increase individual responsibility. What is more disturbing is that standard Western medical thought is sanctioned by our government and by insurance corporations so that significant change from the norm is difficult, if not impossible. We have been conditioned to believe that sickness and health are too complicated for us to comprehend. Only the doctor, with a seemingly "infinite" knowledge, can "cure" us. Any imbalance in our health is seen as sufficient cause to see the doctor. We usually follow our doctor's orders without questions, taking our pills as prescribed. This form of medicine effectively strips individuals of any responsibility for their own sickness or health.

How much do you know about your body and how it works compared to how much you have learned about your external world? Which is more important?

Holistic massage is an expression of the holistic health philosophy. Holistic massage involves two people working together on physical and nonphysical levels to effect positive changes in each. This differs from conventional massage, in which there is a passive receiver who has surrendered responsibility to an active giver who is supposed to have the power to relieve discomfort through direct manipulations. Conventional massage may not be used exclusively as a medium to deal with health problems, but it *always* involves a surrender of responsibility by the receiver. The philosophy and technique of holistic massage are unique because they encourage the receiver to take responsibility for his own state of health. The receiver is an equal and active partner in the massage.

Holistic massage views massage as an art form and strives to stimulate independent thought, self-exploration, and self-discovery in the giver *and* the receiver. Creativity, self-awareness, and an expansion of consciousness are integral parts of holistic massage, and the experiences in this book will allow the reader to discover how these aspects of experience can be gained from any activity.

This book strives to impart to the reader an *understanding* of the basic components of massage and will give you a simple, basic structure to follow. Other massage books offer lengthy descriptions of massage systems, sometimes teaching as many as eighty different strokes. It is more important to understand why something is done rather than trying to memorize detailed descriptions of *what* to do. A technically detailed book forces the reader to memorize a system.

Health care and sick care are moving toward individual responsibility, and this book is an attempt to supply you with vital information you need if you are willing to accept that responsibility. I have been treating sick people for a number of years, and I have found that holistic massage is one of the best and most effective ways to help people help themselves. I have seen myself grow as a result. I would like to share with you what I have learned through practical experience.

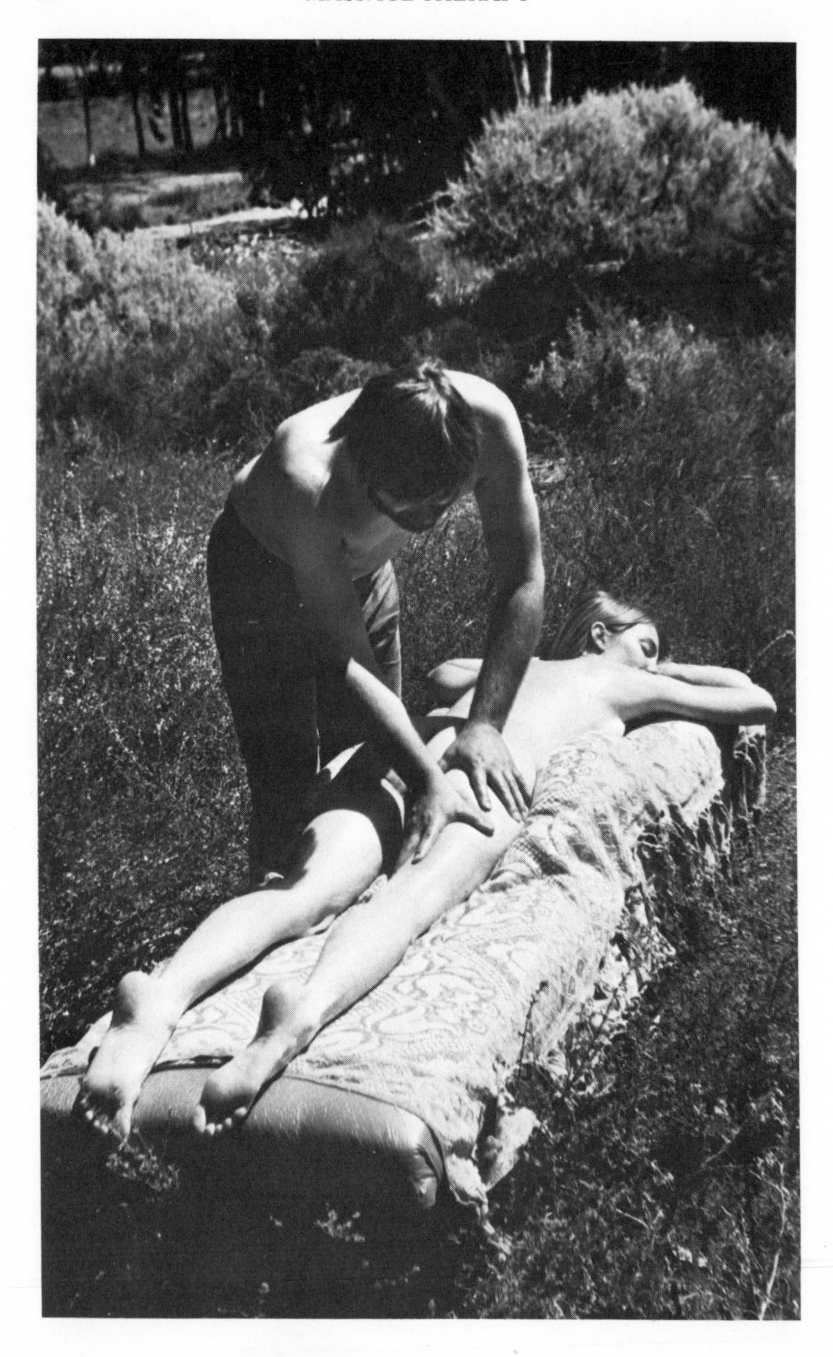

2.

Breathing

Breathing is an important part of holistic massage and health. It is the starting point of all the experiences contained within these pages. The first thing I teach my students is healthy breathing.

There is a yogic saying, "Breath is Life." Without breath, we would die. Air contains oxygen. Every cell in the body requires oxygen more than any other element to sustain life and to carry out its basic functions. Oxygen is carried to the cells by the blood; and the blood, after releasing the life-sustaining oxygen, carries the waste gases back to the lungs to be expelled into the air. The amount of oxygen that gets into the system is directly related to the amount of air that is taken into the lungs with each inhalation. Poor breathing patterns create poor aeration of the lungs, which decreases the body's ability to react to the everyday demands of activity. The body's ability to function healthfully is directly related to the amount of its oxygen intake; therefore, decreased oxygen intake through poor breathing habits decreases the body's capacity to function efficiently.

The lungs almost totally fill the area within the rib cage. There is a flat muscle that is attached to the circumference of the lower ribs. It fits in horizontally between the rib cage and the stomach. This muscle is called the diaphragm and is the major muscle used in proper breathing. The diaphragm is structured to make the lungs work like a set of bellows. This muscle is designed to descend during inhalation, creating a suction effect. In this way, the diaphragm draws air all the way into the lower lobes of the lungs, which are at the bottom of the rib cage, so that the lungs fill from the bottom upwards. After the diaphragm fully descends, the muscles that expand the rib cage are called upon to expand the lungs further, sucking in more air. This descent of the diaphragm causes the stomach to bulge. The whole process should be a naturally occurring, involuntary method of breathing. Unfortunately, most of us have unconsciously learned to breathe differently. I will refer to these unhealthy habits as "chest-type breathing." We actually use our diaphragms in a way opposite to the natural process I have described. In chest-type breathing the diaphragm rises during inhalation, thereby eliminating the bellows effect (see Figure 1). Check your own breathing to see if you have developed these poor habits. The diaphragm suffers from misuse and often disuse, creating a need to relearn healthy breathing patterns. The stomach-in, chest-out philosophy accepted by our public institutions has created a nation of very inhibited breathers.

Experience

The natural way to breathe is called diaphragmatic breathing. Place your hands on your abdomen (stomach area), and notice if they rise or fall while inhaling. If your stomach sucks in during inhalation, you are overusing your chest muscles and losing lung efficiency. Try this: Exhale completely, and as you inhale, try to direct the incoming air all the way into your abdomen so that your hands rise. This may seem very strange at first, but persevere. One common mistake is to try too hard. Breathing should be slow, natural, and very easy. When your abdomen is completely filled, pause for an instant and then let the natural elasticity of the lungs expel the air. At the same time you exhale, allow your muscles to relax and excess tension to leave your body. Keep practicing in a relaxed manner until you get the feel of it. Check your breathing patterns during the day, and soon this healthy, relaxed breathing technique will become a habit.

Chest-type breathing is a natural response to excitement and is a stimulating type of breathing. Diaphragmatic breathing, on the other hand, is a way to calm and relax the body and mind. Use it often.

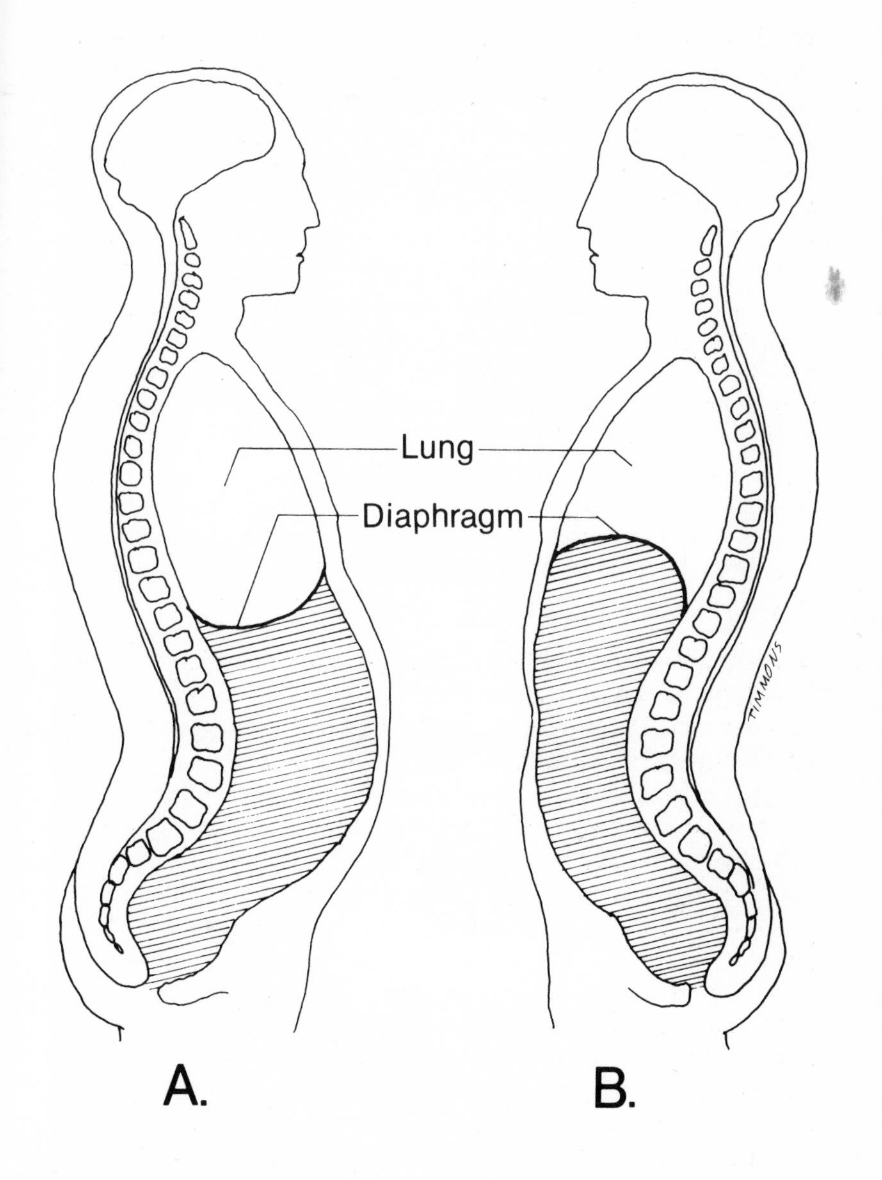

Figure 1. **The Diaphragm.** (A) The diaphragm fully expanded during diaphragmatic inspiration. (B) The diaphragm as it appears during chest-type inspiration. Notice the differences in lung volume.

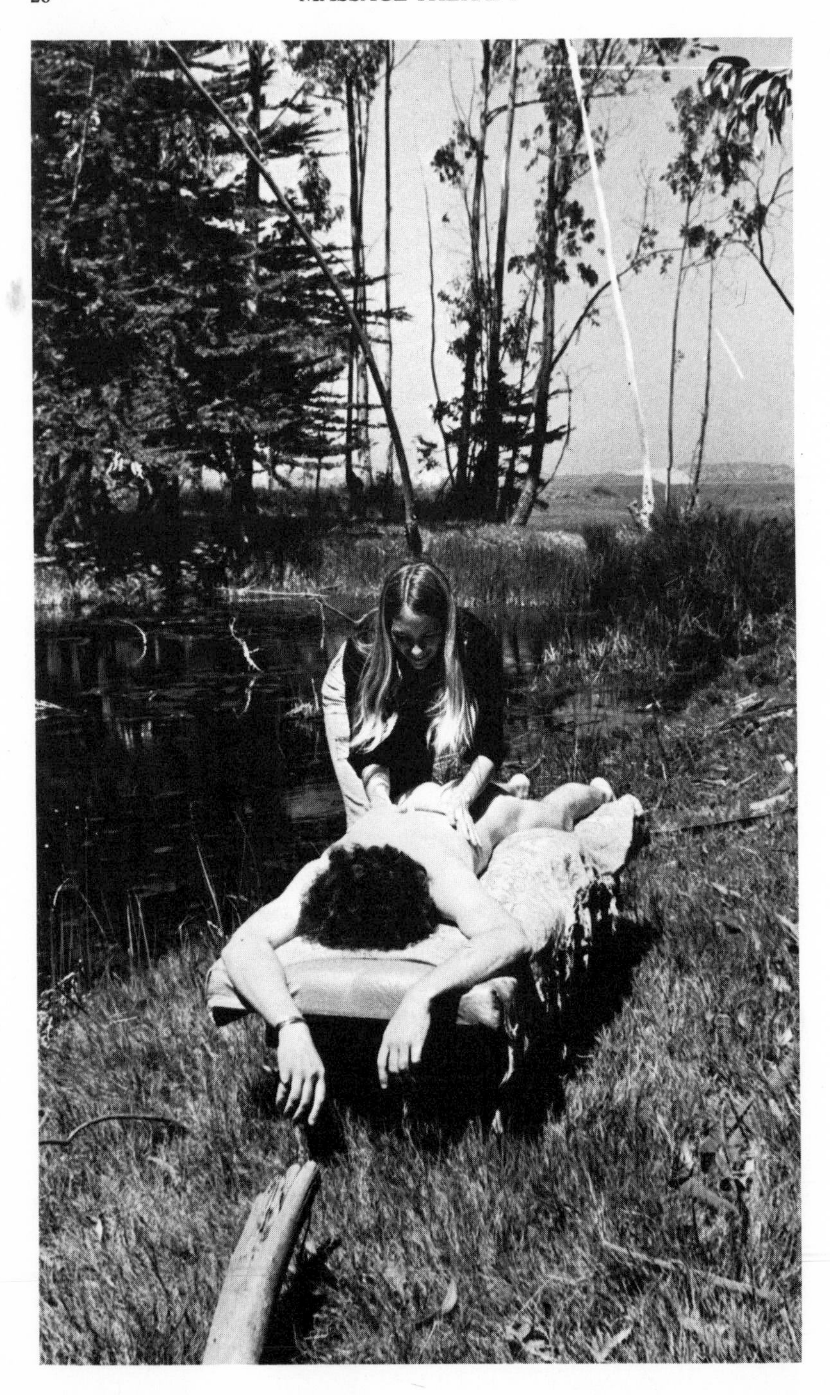

Experience

Rhythmic breathing, or breathing in harmony with your body rhythm (movements), is seldom considered in our physically oriented society. Breathing in harmony with body motion is efficient in terms of strength and energy. To experience this rhythm, stand facing a wall and get into a position as if you were going to push the wall over. First expel all the air in your lungs. Then, as you breathe in, push with all your strength against the wall. Relax for a few breaths. Again, breathe in deeply, and as you exhale, repeat the pushing exercise against the wall. Compare the force you can generate during the inhale push with your strength during the exhale push. Repeat this exercise a few times.

Imagine inhalation as a gathering of energy and strength inward. Exhalation is expressing energy outwards. Movements that require physical effort should be accompanied by exhalation. In holistic massage, as in all types of movement, energy can be controlled and directed through rhythmic breathing. Thus, it is quite important to concentrate on this technique, developing it fully.

Rhythmic breathing is generally conducted by counting to the cadence of your heartbeat. The inhalation to exhalation ratio is approximately 1:2. That is, if the inhalation takes four counts, the exhalation should continue for eight. This is the breathing technique that you will use during holistic massage, patterning your breathing after the rhythm of your body movements. It will help you direct your physical energies, and it also acts to clear your mind so that you can concentrate on the experience at hand. Remember, exhalation should accompany an expression of physical energy whenever possible.

In summary, four types of breathing patterns can be used, depending upon the desired result. There is the shallow, diaphragmatic breath that should be naturally occurring and used throughout the day. Another breath is the deep diaphragmatic breath, which is an excellent way to release tension and calm the body. Then there is the rhythmic breath, which is a deep diaphragmatic breath performed to the inner cadence of the individual; when the rhythmic breath accompanies movement, then the inhalation and exhalation is timed to the physical effort involved. Finally, there is the shallow, chest-type of breath; this is usually the natural response to excitement and should not be used as the normal daily breathing pattern.

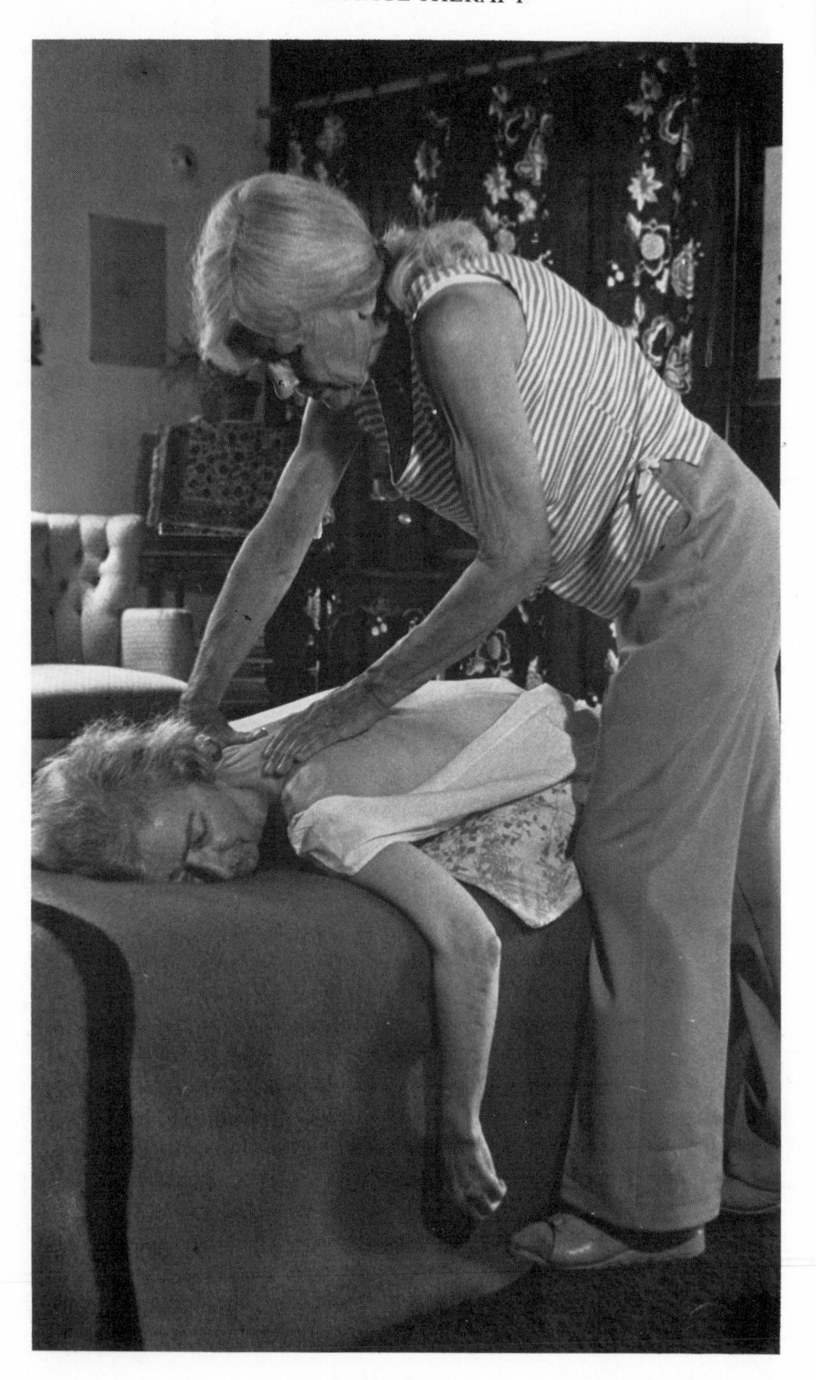

3.

Muscle Tension and Pain

Experience

Find a comfortable position, preferably lying down, and close your eyes. Focus your attention on your head and face and take a deep, diaphragmatic breath. Notice any muscle tension you find there and release this tension as you exhale. When you are finished, your forehead, scalp, face, and jaws should be completely relaxed. Next, focus on your neck and shoulders, making note of any tension. Breathe deeply as before and release the tension on exhalation. Repeat this procedure for each arm, then your chest and abdomen, then your buttocks, thighs, legs, and finally your feet. Take your time and try to gain an inner feeling of your muscles. With each exhalation, allow yourself to relax completely. Think of sinking into the floor and becoming a part of it. The first time you do this relaxation exercise, it should take about thirty minutes to complete.

If you are like most people, you probably found a great deal of tension stored in your body. Nervous tension manifests itself as contracted muscles. We all carry a certain amount of tension within ourselves. Muscle tension in fact is necessary to a degree, because it allows us to remain in a standing position. If you tried to be as relaxed while standing as you were when lying on the floor, you would soon find yourself on the floor again. It takes tension of varying degrees to facilitate body functions. The problem is that most of us have more tension within us than is really necessary. Focus on your shoulders right now. Are they at all tense? How about your forehead or the muscles around your eyes?

Experience

Raise one of your arms overhead. Do it again and again and focus on the amount of effort you exert each time. Next, try to lift your arm using the least amount of muscle tension possible. Notice the difference in energy expenditure. Try to become conscious of how you overuse your body in your daily activities. Often we use many more muscles than needed to get up and down or to move about. A normal body will naturally use a minimum of energy to complete everyday tasks, but many of us get into a habit of using more energy than is necessary. In a sense we override our bodies' natural movement patterns and substitute our own.

Muscles are controlled by nerves. Some muscles are under *voluntary* control, while others react *involuntarily*. Advances in biofeedback have demonstrated that we can learn voluntary control of these involuntary muscles as well. When an impulse is sent down a nerve, the muscle contracts. The degree of *voluntary* muscle contraction can be controlled consciously, as demonstrated in the previous exercise. It is possible to eliminate excess voluntary tension from your body by becoming more conscious of your daily activities and movements. This increased conscious awareness will aid you in reducing muscle tension and wasted energy. Consider the muscle tension caused by involuntary, or unconscious, action. To eliminate this type of tension, we must first explore and understand the ways in which it is formed.

How do you react when you are frightened, angry, frustrated, nervous, or pressured? These emotions cause an unconscious increase in muscle tension, usually relating to the shoulders, face, and upper torso. It also causes shallow, upper-chest breathing patterns.Begin to focus on your shoulders frequently during the day and see how much unnecessary tension you find there. For example, shoulder tension is common while driving a car and is usually unnecessary.

Think back over your life. How did you react to critically emotional experiences? Remember a time when you were really embarrassed, humiliated, or angry? How did you react with your body? Search your past and present and try to recall how your body has reacted to life's most emotional times. If you are like most people, you unconsciously use your body as a shield by tensing your muscles and possibly changing your posture to assume a more defensive attitude. It may be a very minor change in stance, or it may be the way you hold your head or shoulders, but the change occurs. Our tensions and emotional reactions to life situations are determined very early in life. But these are not necessarily the best ways to cope with stress.

We are all deceivers to one degree or another, if not verbally, then emotionally. What do you do when you feel an emotion while relating to another person but would rather not have that person perceive your reaction? I find myself holding the emotion back by tensing my muscles. This tensing of my muscles is subtle enough that my friend does not realize the existing tension. Nevertheless, that tension does exist, and my response is a learned response. I learned long ago in similar situations that my response produced a successful result, and I probably will continue to use that response unconsciously as long as I continue to be successful with it.

Sometimes we have an unconscious fear of expressing our emotions in a natural way—a conditioned response carried over from early childhood. Again let your mind wander into the past and try to remember how very natural, healthy emotional outbursts were handled by your parents. If your family was like mine and most others, I would guess that natural outbursts that your parents saw as inappropriate were swiftly suppressed with a slap, a cold stare, a threat, or—most effective of all—a withdrawal of love. All children are subject to conditioning, just as Pavlov conditioned dogs. Rewards are given for responses deemed appropriate by those in control, not necessarily for natural responses. It is my sincere hope that some of the techniques presented in this book will help you decondition yourself so that you can achieve more natural emotional and bodily responses to a variety of life situations.

Suppression of emotions is a voluntary response. Repression of emotions results from voluntary suppression that has become unconscious habit. It should be apparent from the previous discussion that each response to stress involves an increase in muscle tension. Emotions are actually stored in the body in the form of chronic muscle tension and are a primary cause of headaches, back pain, and poor posture. Common slang, such as "uptight," is often very accurate and perceptive. If we repress emotions, we get uptight. Our muscles tense, and the natural energy flow of our bodies is obstructed. Emotions are like rivers. There are rapids and areas of calm, flowing water. There are unpredictable bends, and the course of the river is likely to change many times throughout its lifetime. If the flow is obstructed by a dam, it does not stop the flow completely. Water still rushes in. The water backs up, floods the surrounding countryside, and forms a reservoir which also needs to be controlled. If the water is not controlled, it might burst the dam, and such a release will cause far more damage to the countryside than if the river had been left unimpeded by a dam. Emotions, like rivers, need unobstructed flow. Just because you dam them up does not mean you will stop the incoming flow, and your restraint is not going to make them go away. They will just continue to amass until you deal with them. Emotions need to be experienced without inhibitions and then released and allowed to flow through.

Another aspect to consider when dealing with muscle tension is posture. Posture affects muscle tension, and muscle tension affects posture. Normal upright posture (see Figure 2) is an alignment of the body against the pull of gravity that requires the least amount of energy and muscle tension to be maintained. This position is one in which a vertical line drawn down the side of the body will pass through the ear lobe, shoulder, hip, knee, and ankle. *Minor* variations are to be expected. But when the body is out of alignment, it begins to work against the downward pull of gravity. This causes an increased expenditure of energy through the increased muscle contraction necessary to hold the body upright.

Emotions cause muscle tensions which affect posture. Muscles are made of fibers which run parallel to one another, and the fibers are made of filaments (see Figure 3). The ends of muscles are called tendons, and these are attached to bones (see Figure 4). When a muscle contracts, it pulls one bone toward another, creating movement. This explains how emotions affect posture. Emotions cause an increase in nervous tension, which in turn causes an increase in muscle tension. When tension increases, the position of the body is bound to change by the very action of muscles pulling on bone. These changes are imperceptible at first, but each change adds to previous changes, resulting in very distorted body posture and concomitant increased tension. When the body is out of vertical alignment, the force of gravity will cause it to topple over unless muscles are contracted to hold the person upright. Over the years, muscle tension becomes deep-seated, and the corresponding change in posture becomes ingrained.

Our posture also changes as we mimic the attitudes and postures of others we admire. Humans learn by imitating others. If our parents have poor posture, we may develop the same bad

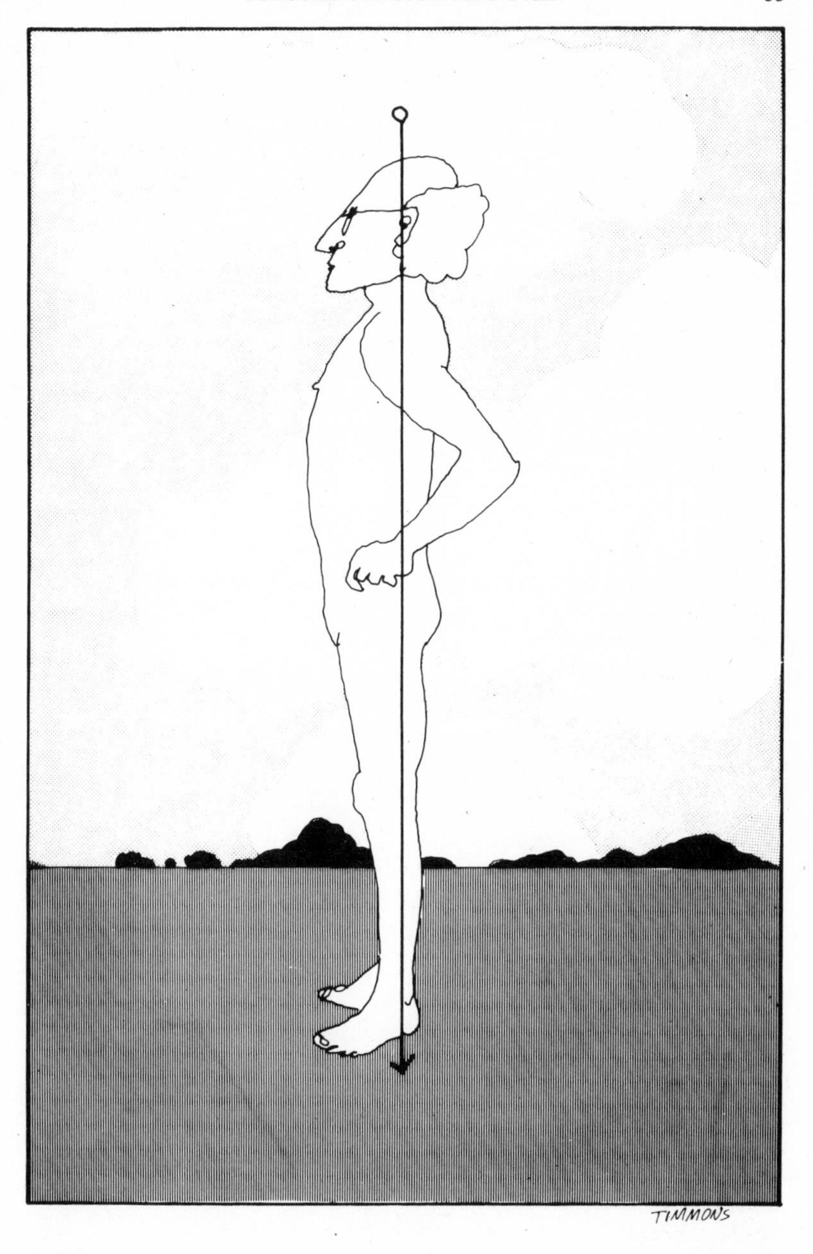

Figure 2. **"Normal" Posture.** An imaginary vertical line drawn down the side should pass through the earlobe, shoulder, hip, knee, and just in front of the ankle joint.

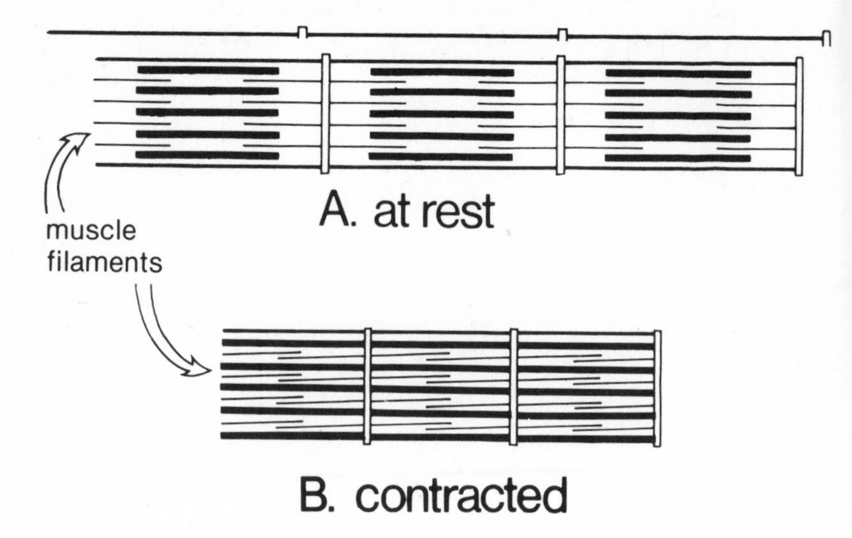

Figure 3. **Muscle Fiber.** (A) A muscle fiber at rest as viewed through an electron microscope. Notice that the muscle fiber is made of filaments. (B) A fully contracted muscle fiber. The filaments slide together.

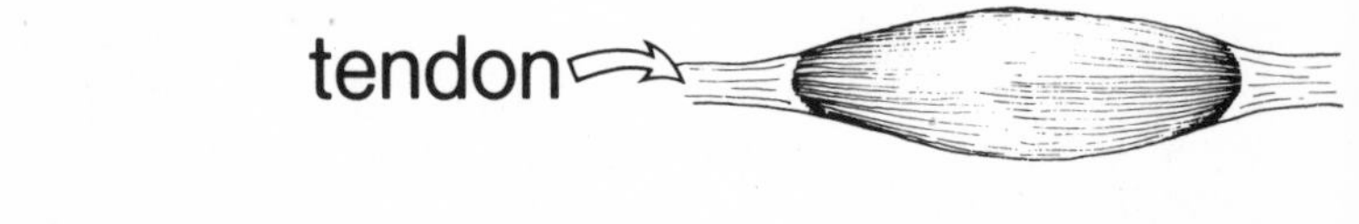

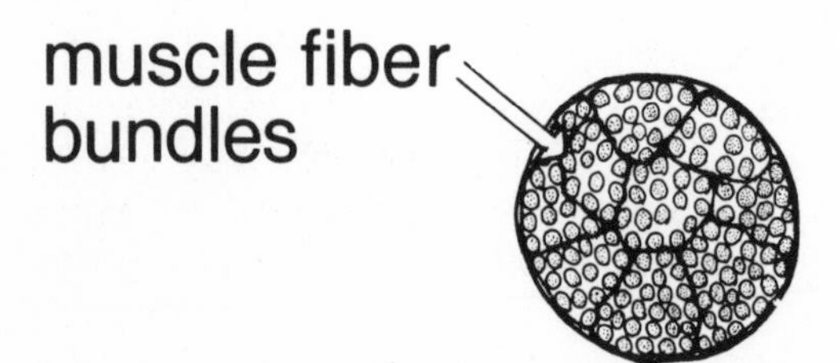

Figure 4. **Muscle Belly.** This shows a muscle belly tapering into tendons of attachment. A cross-section of the muscle belly reveals bundles of muscle fibers.

habits. Sometimes we imitate actors or actresses who may have poor posture. What looks good on the screen may be completely unnatural in reality. Some people believe the stance of a model to be particularly sexy or attractive and try to imitate it. In our adolescent years we are most vulnerable. Females have the problem of overdeveloped or underdeveloped breasts. They sometimes assume a caved-in chest posture, an unnatural stance which is almost certain to cause back and neck problems in later life. Too, there is the male or female who assumes the chest-out, shoulders-back posture that will be a source of back pain later on in life. Faulty posture is a learned response that causes muscle tension. The new body attitudes become involuntary, and muscle tension becomes ingrained. Such unnecessary tension is bound to cause pain eventually.

The important thing to understand is that the whole process involves conscious, learned responses that soon progress to involuntary habits. When emotions are suppressed and repressed during life, and as posture changes in response to this, muscle tension results in chronic spasms which in turn cause pain. The best way to deal with this cycle is through holistic massage and exercises in self-awareness.

Holistically, emotional tension can be seen as an imbalance of a person's mental or spiritual aspects causing physical symptoms of muscle tension and pain. Massage alone or even hot baths with massage will not permanently affect the condition. The mental and spiritual attitudes must be changed by the individual through self-awareness and conscious effort before there can be permanent physical change. The first and most difficult step is for the individual to realize that pain reveals an imbalance. All of us like to think that we are mentally and spiritually balanced. If that were true, our physical bodies would also be in balance. If it is not, something is wrong, and the first step toward correcting the problem lies in admitting that fact to one's self. You may then be able to realize what is causing the imbalance or disharmony. Much sickness is the result of blocked energy flow or unexpressed action outwardly manifested as stress. When you are able to get in touch with the original action, emotion, or feeling and thereby unblock the flow, the problem may be resolved. The emotion, tension, posture, or pain syndrome that can block a person's energy flow is a result of that person's perception of, and reaction to, his environment. These perceptions are based on mental and spiritual attitudes about one's self, others, and one's surroundings. I suggest changes in basic attitudes and body-use habits to effect changes in the physical condition.

Muscle tension is not the only cause of pain. There are other obvious sources of pain with which we are all familiar. Muscular and ligamentous strain are two of the prime causes of body aches and pains. Muscles that are underused and then abused will always become sore and tense. Muscles are also subject to tears and bruises that may result from direct blows. These are all familiar, common problems that may seem very simple to understand. My experience as a physical therapist, however, has made me look behind the obvious and try to see how common aches and pains relate to stored muscle tension or mind/body/spirit imbalance.

The body faces its greatest danger of injury when subjected to an uncontrolled movement. A common injury treated in physical therapy offices is whiplash. This most often results from a rear-end collision in which the occupants of the first car sustain an uncontrolled snap of their heads and necks. My experience has been that the most severe cases of whiplash were sustained by people who seemed to have been out of harmony emotionally. This is not to say that all whiplash victims are neurotic. Rather, I have found that the worst cases were people I would have expected to find loaded with chronic tension just by observing their personality characteristics. Muscle tension causes poor flexibility, which increases the severity of a traumatic injury. The same applies to chronic back pain. People with chronic back pain very often exhibit poor flexibility. And until the inflexibility is changed, along with the attitudes and habits that caused the inflexibility, the back pain will continue to recur.

Another example of body/mind/spirit imbalance is provided by weekend athletes, those individuals who rest during the week and then participate in vigorous sports on their days off. There are basic imbalances within the body/mind/spirit complex of the weekend athlete that Monday morning pains are trying to communicate to the individual. Most of us suffer from the mental attitude that we can be dormant for five or more days and then be hyperactive for one or two. Common sense should tell us this will not work, but we nevertheless continue with the unbalanced activity. There is a spiritual imbalance in the weekend athlete, a spiritual irreverence for the body. The body cannot be abused through disuse, followed by misuse. A person who has a spiritual reverence for his body will feed it the correct amount of food and exercise to keep it optimally healthy. Such a body will respond to any reasonable demand placed upon it.

The *causes* of aches and pains are much deeper than most of us have previously considered. An individual does not suffer a sore arm because he throws a ball too hard. The real cause lies within a complex of attitudes and beliefs held by that individual. One set of attitudes allowed the arm to become inflexible and weak through limited use. Another set of attitudes led the individual to the athletic field without properly conditioning his body first. Yet another set of attitudes caused him to try to throw a ball much harder than he was capable of doing. In short, the pain has not been caused by torn muscles so much as it has been caused by a group of attitudes and beliefs held by the individual.

The long-term results of stored tension are numerous and, in many cases, very serious. We need to learn and practice better ways of handling life's tensions before damage to the body is irreparable. Long-term, permanent change happens within the individual. A doctor or masseur cannot take a problem involving tension away from another person. It is the individual's responsibility; only he can secure long-term changes in his own body.

As you practice massage, your hands will develop a keen sense for locating muscle tension and spasm. It is the responsibility of the giver to point out these areas to the receiver and explore with him the possible reasons for the excess tensions. Remember, only the receiver can really know the true cause of his tension, and only he can eliminate it. Holistic massage is structured so that the receiver will focus on his tensions, but sometimes he is reluctant to investigate possible sources of his tensions. That is why the giver should initiate and encourage discussion about what he has found. He can sometimes draw out thoughts and feelings from the receiver that otherwise might be left buried. Some of the greatest benefits holistic massage has to offer occur during the period of reflection directly following the massage.

Experience

Holistic massage and self-awareness are helpful in dealing with muscle tension. Much of our tension is caused by blocked emotions, so additional exercises in releasing those emotions can be helpful and fun.

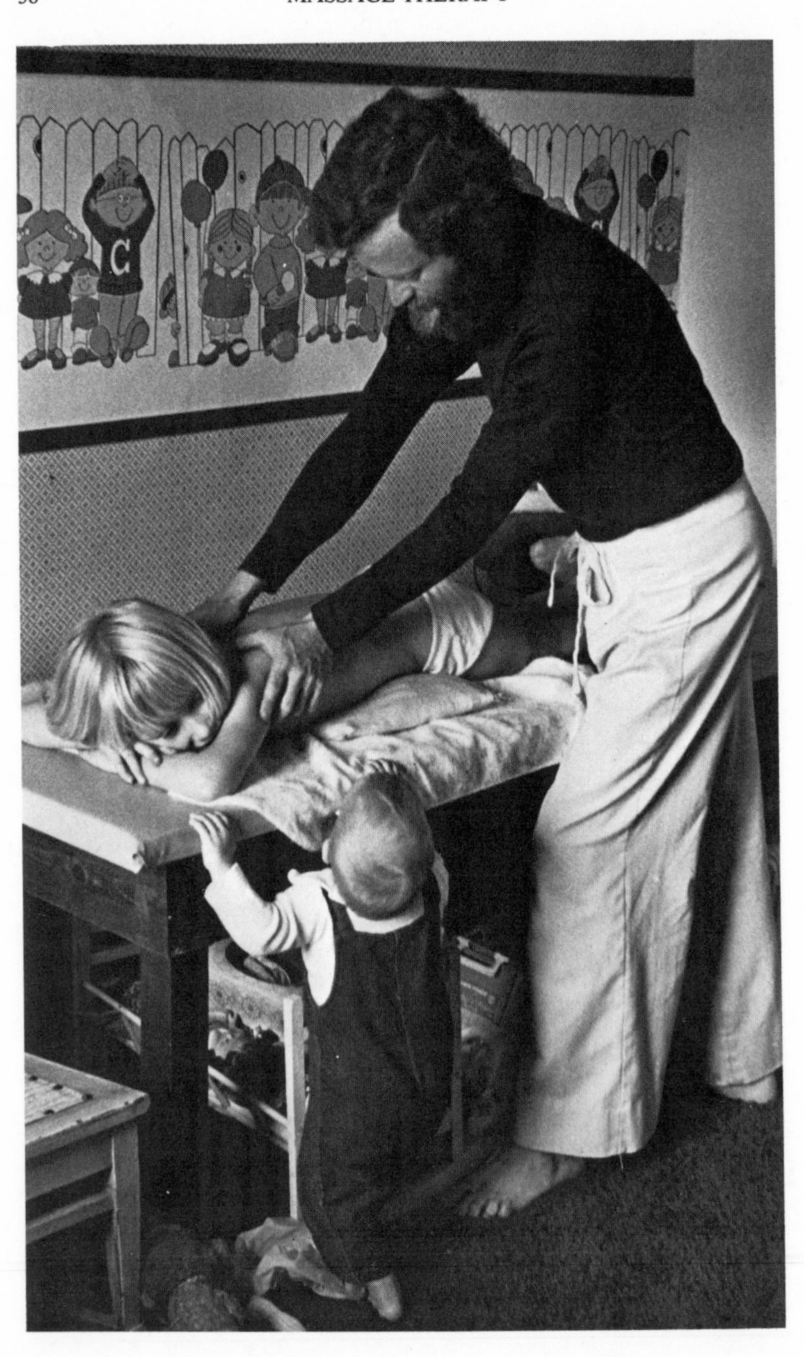

Have you ever taken a tennis racquet, broom, or any such device and attacked your bed? It may sound absurd, but everyone has experienced relief from anger, frustration, or tension by expending physical energy. This exercise is much safer than throwing a glass against the wall or kicking a hole in the door. Beating on a bed is just as effective, and it will not cost you a cent in damages. When you are really tense or angry, let yourself go and follow your emotions. Shout, laugh, cry—do anything that feels natural. Sometimes when I am angry and driving in a car (alone, of course), I find myself screaming and yelling, and eventually I feel a lot better for it.

When you finish these exercises, try to rest your mind on positive thoughts. Feel good about yourself and your health. Develop a positive image and a feeling of well-being.

Muscle tension causing acute or chronic pain and poor postural attitudes is usually deep-seated and difficult to deal with. The causes of the tension are not usually clearly defined. Many aspects of a person's life come together, or coalesce, to create that person's health at any given moment. This book is filled with numerous experiences which will enable you to explore various aspects of your own life. In this way, you can search for your own answers regarding the formation of muscle tension. There are also many exercises that will help you deal more effectively with your own tensions and everyday aches and pains. This is all part of the holistic philosophy, which prescribes individual responsibility.

Two factors are of primary importance when searching for your own mental/physical/spiritual attitudes contributing to those particular tensions and pains. First, be honest with yourself. Avoid both overestimation and underestimation of your problems. Some people completely deny physical tensions or refuse to take any responsibility for them, and others tend to chastise or denigrate themselves for having so much tension. Secondly, try to realize that reducing tensions or eliminating aches and pains often involves a very long and concentrated effort. Good health is, in fact, a never-ending process. Use the exercises in this book to start on the road to better health.

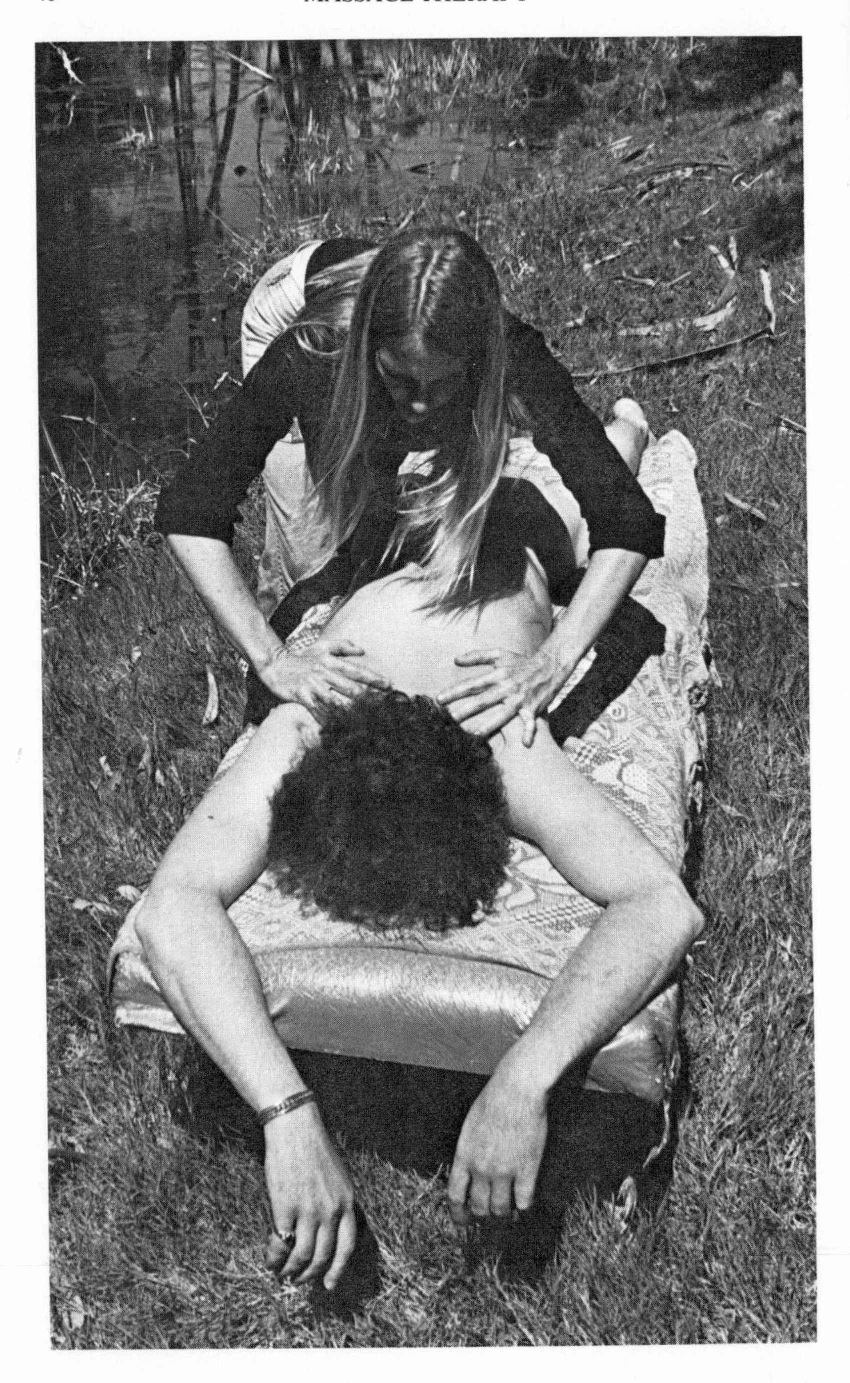

4.

The Body as an Energy System

Western practitioners have always viewed the body as a solid, physical mass with the skin marking its outer boundaries. For centuries, specialized medical science has seen the body as an island unto itself. This view isolates us from our true relationship with the environment and tends to make us believe that human beings operate under a different set of laws than the rest of creation. The holistic approach, on the other hand, considers the body as a dynamic energy system that is in a constant state of change and that is directly affected by changes in the environment, social conditions, mental attitudes, and personal habits.

This new view of medicine draws from both ancient and modern sources. Our empirical, scientific methodology cannot prove or disprove the validity of the new medicine, because the old methodology lacks the technology to research and test the basic assumptions of the holistic approach. It is nearly impossible to research a philosophy, and the new medicine is based more on philosophy than on that which researchers feel is valid Western science. The new medicine considers lasting results more important than methodology.

The view of the body as a dynamic energy system is best understood and validated by blending the ancient philosophy of acupuncture with modern theories of quantum mechanics. Modern physics views the universe as energy in motion and in a constant state of change. These radical and enlightening concepts were born in the minds of men such as Einstein, Louis Victor de Broglie, and Max Planck. Each said that all matter is composed of a basic energy essence, designated as light energy. Your body, the ground you walk on, this book, and everything else in the universe are the same in this basic sense. Everything is composed of waves of electromagnetic light energy. We are not solid at all. It just appears that way. The body is actually a swirling, dynamic ball of electromagnetic energy that has a flow of energy and properties of polarity. This means we have positive and negative poles and that our physical structure follows the laws of electricity and magnetism.

I could use the same words and concepts to describe the philosophy of acupuncture. Acupuncture is a philosophy with roots in ancient Taoist thought. This, like quantum mechanics, views the universe as being composed of one primal energy. Ultimately, there is only the eternal Tao. Tao is a gestalt of two aspects: yin and yang. This is often referred to as negative and positive. However, it really means much more than these words imply. Yin and yang encompass all duality—female and male, out and in, receptive and expressive, up and down, and so on. These aspects are not separated as we often assume. They are inseparable parts of the one eternal Tao. Everything is energy, yin and yang, and together they are Tao. Man and his environment are one. They coexist as members of an ancient family that cannot be dissolved.

Flowing within the body are currents of energy that the orientals call Ki. This concept is compatible with the postulates or laws of modern physics, which state that if something has the property of polarity, then it must have a current flow. Ki energy flows throughout the body along meridians. Figure 5 shows the main acupuncture meridians. When there is an imbalance or blockage of Ki energy—which is also to say there is an imbalance of yin and yang—then illness can result. There is an energy imbalance long before a symptom manifests itself physically. The Eastern approach to treating an illness consists of two parts. One approach is to balance the energy flow by stimulating points along the energy meridians. The second approach is to interview the patient about his thoughts, habits, attitudes, and so on. This helps the acupuncturist determine the *cause* of the energy imbalance. The physical body is not segregated from psychological or spiritual considerations, and Taoist philosophy does not allow the segregation of the body and its environment. It is all Tao. The important point here is that if the cause of the imbalance is not discovered and eliminated, then the treatment will not be effective.

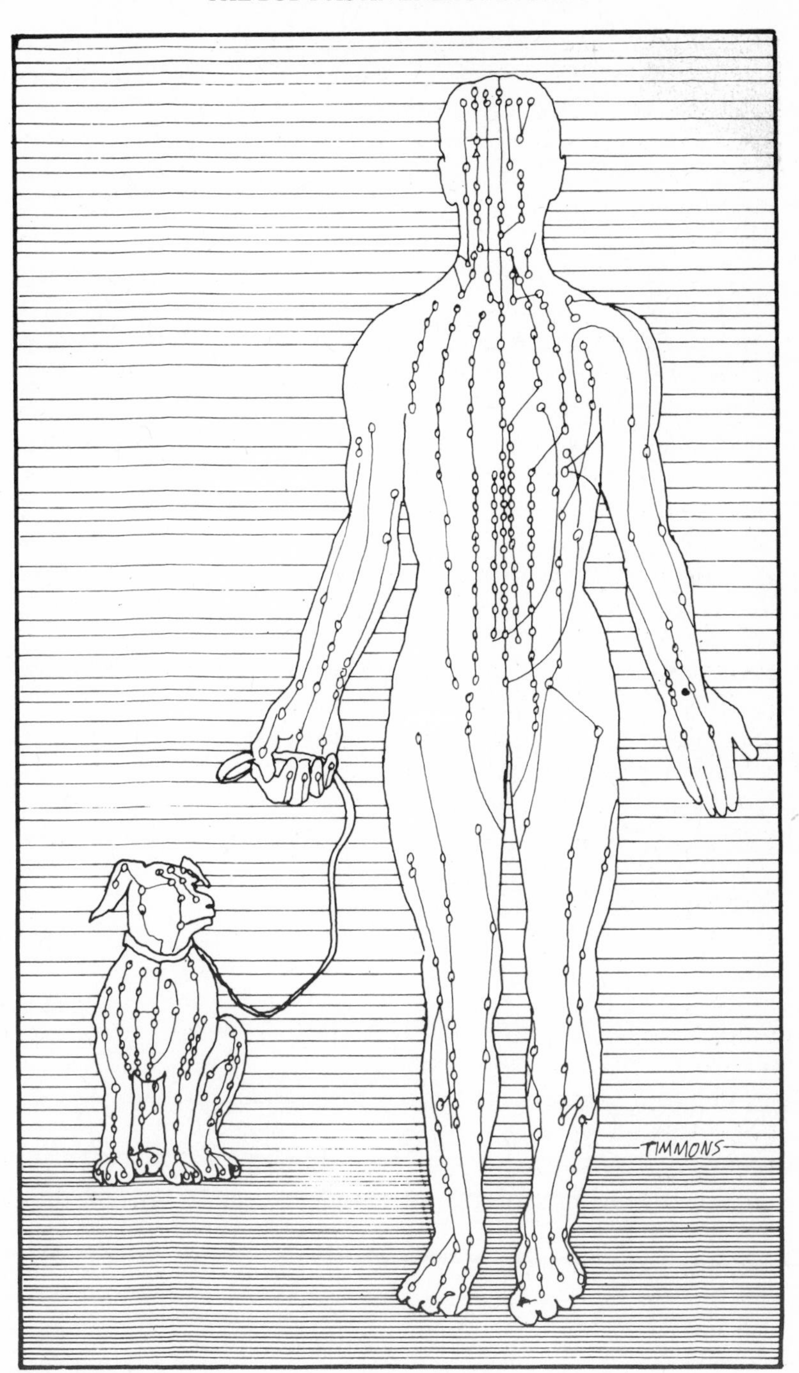
TIMMONS

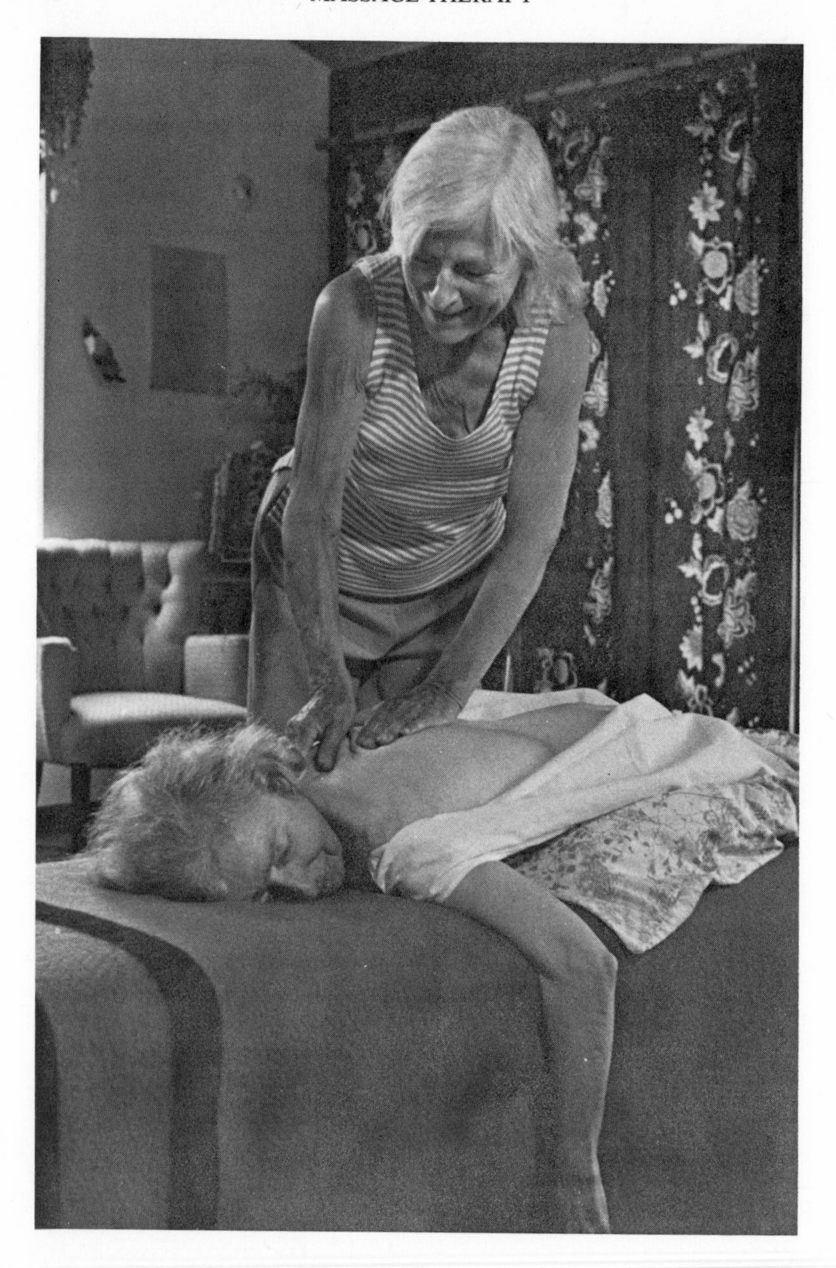

The holistic view that all of life is an interdependent, dynamic energy system is supported by more than modern physics and ancient philosophies. Modern researchers are beginning to study and acknowledge the idea that man, the whole being, is intimately related to his environment. For example, there is mounting evidence that 70 to 90 percent of all cancer is linked to environmental causes. We are literally killing ourselves and our planet through abuse and pollution. Too, we are beginning to understand that personal habits—mental, physical, and spiritual—are more important to health than any other factors regarding sickness, health, or healing.

My purpose in discussing these matters is twofold. First, I am trying to stimulate you to consider the body in terms other than those with which we have been brought up. Second, I want you to appreciate some potential healing benefits of massage that are not generally considered.

Many healing arts are gaining acceptance today that are based in Taoist philosophy and do not require needles, as does acupuncture. Energy imbalances can be treated by many forms of stimulation of the points along the energy meridians. This includes stimulation by pressure that is applied by hands and fingers. Massage can help balance the energy flow of the body, because many of the manipulations stimulate the energy points and thereby increase energy flow. Massage is useful as a preventative measure as well as an aid to cure. Holistic massage is a natural process in which two people work together to improve their states of health—mental, physical, and spiritual.

I encourage you to look at the body as a dynamic energy system, one which is intimately related to the environment, whose health or illness is under far greater individual control than we have ever dreamed possible. Maybe we even have *total* control.

A good place to begin experiencing the body as an energy system is with an exploration into body-awareness exercises. These will start you on the road to greater self-awareness—*the* most important aspect of holistic health and massage.

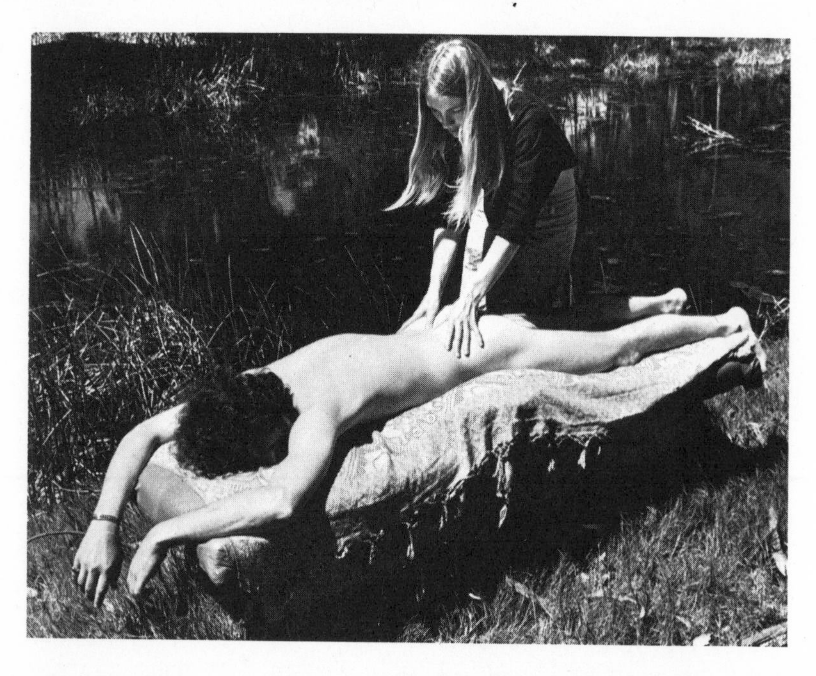

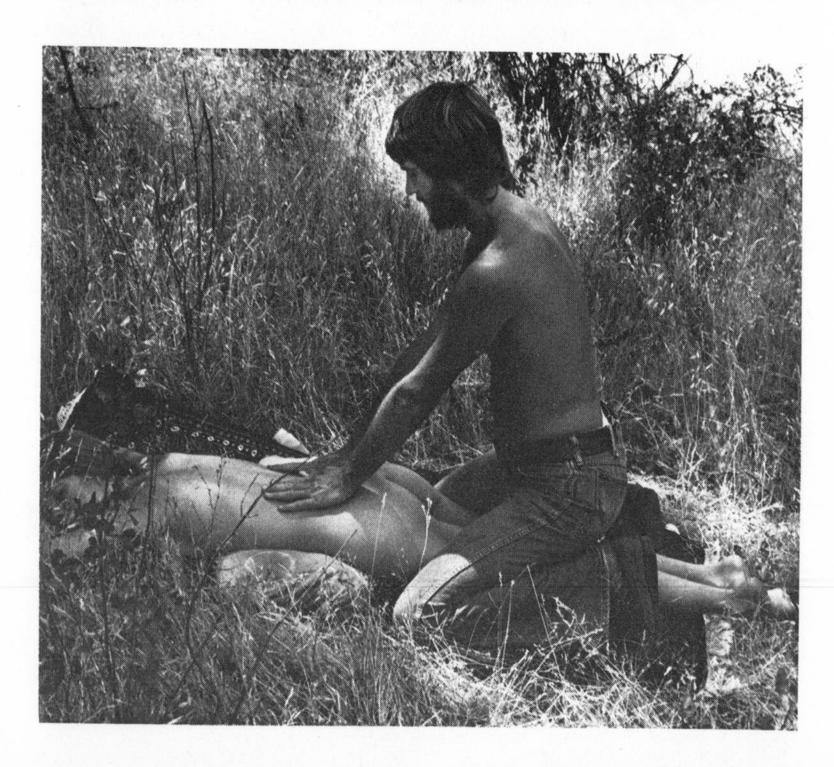

5.

Body Awareness

Experience

Close your eyes and turn your attention to your lower left leg. Can you sense the presence of your leg? If you have a definite feel for your leg, try to feel it in detail. Can you sense the full surfaces of your foot: top, bottom, and sides? Can you sense all around your ankle and lower leg? Next, concentrate on the other parts of your body, taking one segment at a time. Determine which areas you can feel or sense clearly and which areas are "dead," or lacking feeling. Some areas may feel distorted in size or shape. Pay special attention to your joints. When you have focused on all of the body segments in turn, see if you can sense your total body image. Some areas may feel enlarged; others may feel constricted. You may sense one side of your body completely differently from the other side. An area which has been the source of constant problems throughout life may feel quite distorted. Make a mental note of which areas of your body are sensually "dead" and which are distorted.

Body awareness is a sense, just like our other senses. But unlike the "outer" senses of sight, smell, taste, hearing, and touch, we cannot determine with certainty the exact mechanism that causes us to sense our bodies. However, partial explanation lies in sense receptors located in the skin, muscles, and joints.

Sense receptors are specialized structures that are stimulated by changes in the environment or changes within the body. Stimulation of a receptor results in an electrical message that is sent along nerve fibers to the spinal cord and brain where the message is decoded, analyzed, and perceived as sensation. Receptors are classified according to the stimulus to which they respond. Thus, there are receptors of touch, heat, cold, pain, vibration, and movement.

Mechano-receptors (the receptors of movement) respond to changes in muscle or bone position and are important, in conjunction with the other types of receptors, in giving us body awareness. The brain correlates all data from the various sense receptors, and the result is body sense. This is the theory used by the medical profession to explain body awareness.

There is a phenomenon, however, that has been puzzling people for generations, and it cannot be ignored in a discussion of body awareness. This phenomenon is called "phantom limb." When a person has a part of his body amputated, he continues to be "aware" of the lost part, to have the illusion that it is still there. For instance, if someone loses a leg, he continues to sense the leg. He can sense it move, can wiggle his toes, and unfortunately, he can sometimes sense pain. These are cases of body awareness without the body. Disturbing questions begin to arise. How can body position, heat, cold, and pain be sensed without sense receptors? Are there other aspects of sensory awareness that we have ignored for lack of an explanation but that can someday be scientifically verified? Remember, the philosophy of acupuncture cannot yet be verified scientifically, although its therapeutic benefits are widely recognized.

To be fair to present-day medical science, I must point out that the generally accepted theory of phantom limb is that the ends of the nerves at the amputation site are randomly sending sensory messages to the brain. This may seem to be a plausible explanation, but a closer examination raises some doubts regarding its validity. I have described to you how sensory messages originate (by stimulation of highly specialized sense receptors), and the scientific explanation of phantom limb does not make clear how sensory impulses can originate from the end of an amputated nerve, where few, if any, sense receptors exist. It is like saying that a telegraph office that sends messages along wires is not really needed in sending the messages—the wires can do it on their own if the telegraph office is destroyed.

Phantom limb, like acupuncture, cannot be adequately explained by scientists, because (1) they consider the body only as a

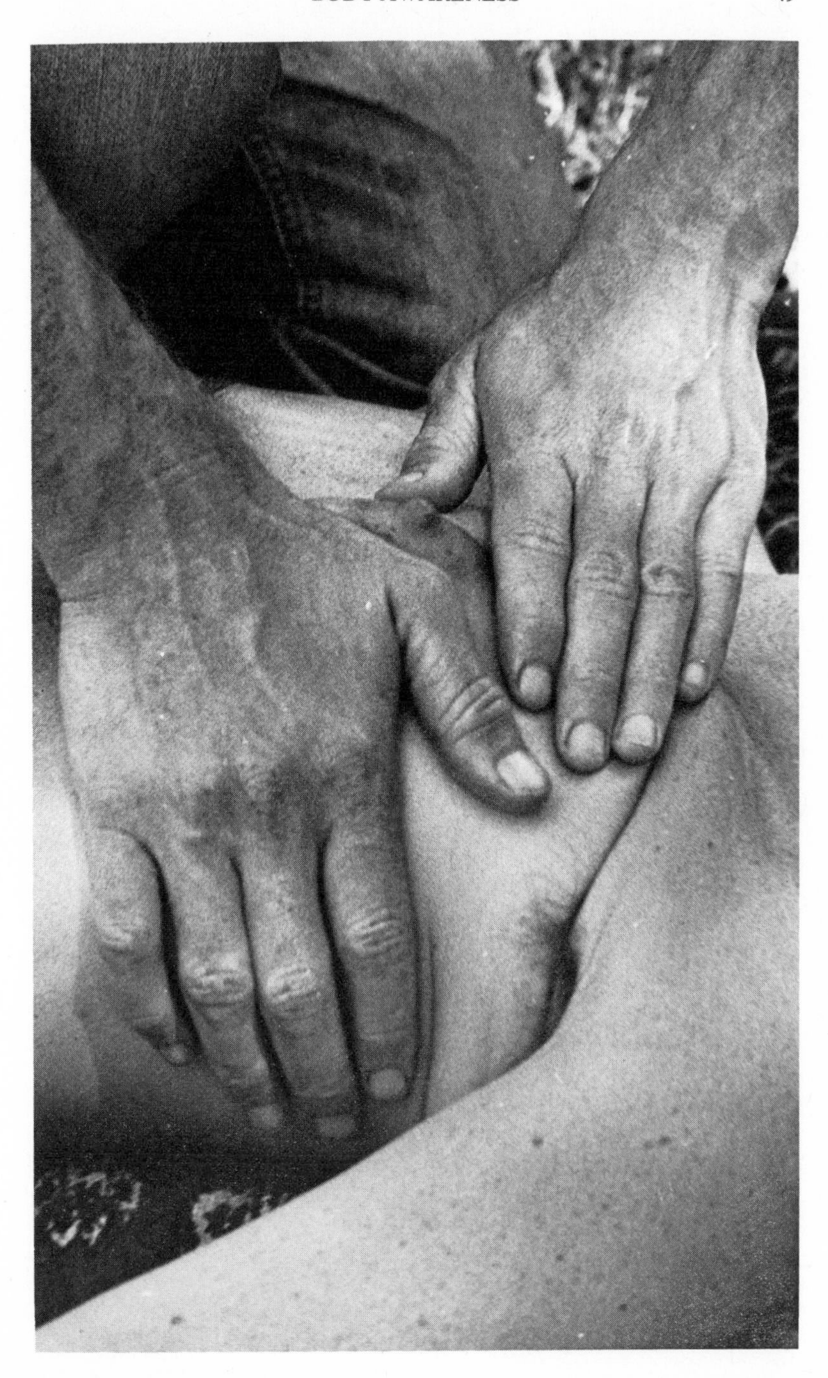

physical structure and not as an electromagnetic energy system and (2) present technology does not permit objective study of the body as an energy system.

There is reason to believe that body awareness is the result of two sensory systems. The physical sensory system, as previously described, informs the conscious mind of the physical body's states of being and change. The energy counterpart of the physical body can be referred to as the energy body. As discussed in Chapter 4, our bodies are complex, electromagnetic systems, and our energies thus extend beyond our skins in characteristic patterns, like the electromagnetic patterns of a bar magnet. Just because we cannot visually perceive the energy body does not mean that it does not exist. This body appears to have a sensory feedback mechanism that tells the conscious mind of the energy body's state of being and change. Such a view not only takes us a long way toward a comprehensive understanding of phantom limb; it also shows the importance of body awareness in health and healing.

Phantom limb may be an expression of the energy body. Evidence to support this theory has come from advances in high-voltage Kirlean photography. Kirlean photography appears to demonstrate the existence of an energy aura surrounding a variety of objects, including the human body. A phenomenon called phantom leaf has been observed. A Kirlean photograph of a normal leaf shows a normal aura. If a portion of the leaf is torn away, the aura remains. Research is still being conducted on Kirlean photography because many questions remain unanswered. But so far, Kirlean photography gives convincing evidence, though not conclusive, that the body is an electromagnetic energy system. The phantom leaf photographs lend evidence to the theory that phantom limb and its accompanying sensations are an expression of the energy body.

The physical and energy bodies are joined as one, but they are not inseparable. Each has the property of sensory feedback to tell the mind the true state of the body. Scientists have always viewed sensations as coming exclusively from the physical system. But have you ever experienced pain or other sensations that simply do not have physical origins? Scientists explain this phenomenon by referring to it as pain or sensation of a "nonspecific origin." I believe these sensations originate in the energy body and that they can provide us with information in a positive and healthful way.

Body awareness is helpful in locating areas of tension, pain, and blocked energy and can help you learn to sense energy flow. Difficulties in achieving body awareness can also be helpful in locating areas of our bodies that we have completely denied. These are the "dead" areas to which I referred earlier. Variations in body awareness can indicate areas of imbalanced energy flow. As stated in the philosophies of acupuncture and Shiatsu (acupressure), an imbalance of the flow of energy will eventually cause disease, and a balancing of these energies will benefit health. It is possible to use holistic massage and visual imagery to help balance and align your own energy flow. You will also increase your self-awareness.

Re-Membering

A few years ago I was visiting institutions for the blind and studying some of the methods they were using to increase body awareness and body image. At one school I saw the results of a very revealing study on body image. Each student in a select group was given a ball of clay and asked to mold it into the shape of his body. The results pointed to a difference between body awareness and full body image. Not one clay figure was whole. Sometimes an arm was missing, or a leg or one or more extremities was out of place or not even connected to the body proper. Most heads were separated from the torso. Some arms were huge, and others were small. There was not one model that demonstrated symmetry or equally proportioned extremities. The blind students certainly had an awareness of body parts, but they definitely had very distorted body images.

Sighted people, on the other hand, have the benefit of visual feedback to tell them that the body is whole. Faced with the task of modeling our body images out of clay, we would naturally fashion the body as a whole piece. The gift of sight is misleading in this case, however, because we may not actually *feel* whole.

At the beginning of this chapter, I suggested you close your eyes and try to become aware of your individual body parts. Then, I asked you to try to sense your total body image. In most cases, a person naturally senses his body as a whole, because his sight has told him for years that it could not be any other way. Think back to when you concentrated on each separate part of your body. Did you find any dead spots? Were any joints perceived as "dead" spots? If your answer to either of these questions is yes, then you could not possibly sense your full body image as a whole.

An incomplete body image indicates distorted awareness. It is common to have preconceived ideas and beliefs that obscure perception and awareness. The young blind students came up with distorted body images that were accurate reflections of their perceptions. Try the body-awareness exercises again with the realization that it is not abnormal to have a distorted body image.

Gaps in body image usually occur in joints and on the back of the body. The areas we do not see or touch often are the most difficult to sense. When I started working on my own body image, I was amazed at how many "dead" areas I had. The more I tried to sense my body as a whole, the more distorted my image became. In my search for an honest body image, I became more and more perceptive of daily and weekly changes in my body. I became much more sensitive to my inner environment and to how it changes with the days and weeks.

Holistic massage is an effective way to increase body awareness and to become more familiar with the inner environment of the body. Emphasis is placed on the receiver becoming consciously aware of his body and body image. This is especially effective for the "dead" areas over the back of the body. Massage stimulates each part, or member, of the body so that it is possible to "re-member" the body. Bringing together the separate members of the body and gaining a full body image is helpful in dealing with areas of energy blockage, imbalance, and possible health problems. The full body sense is a sense that needs conscious development.

Experience

In order to re-member the body, it is important to gain an inner sense of the body's energy flows. You can try the following exercise to gain a sense of your own energies. Lie down on the floor and close your eyes. Focus on your right arm until you get an image or awareness of it. Do the same with your left arm and then compare the two. Get a clear feeling of how one compares to the other. Next, squeeze one hand very hard for ten to fifteen seconds. Release, and repeat this exercise. Bend your wrist back for ten to fifteen seconds. Release, and then repeat. Next, contract your upper arm as hard as possible by bending your elbow. Again, release and repeat. Now compare your awareness of one arm to the other. How do your arms feel now compared to how they matched up before? They may feel of different size and weight. See if you perceive other ways in which they differ. There are, of course, definite physical changes. Part of what you are sensing are physical body messages caused by muscle contraction and variations in arm circulation. It is the sensations *apart from* the physical body on which you should focus. What are the sensations outside of your skin, surrounding your arm? There are definite sensations perceived around the physical body extending quite a distance into space. This exercise can be repeated for different parts of your body to increase your sense of body awareness and energy flow. It can be very helpful when trying to learn what an imbalance between body halves feels like. As body energies are freed through massage, body parts may feel lighter, warmer, or larger. Try these exercises again and again, and soon you will begin to "re-member" what you lost or maybe never had.

As you explore body awareness and gain a truer body image, you will become familiar with areas that are tense, distorted, or "dead." Pinpoint these areas and then ask yourself why they feel the way they do. Here, again, the key to benefiting from holistic massage and the awareness exercises is your active participation. Do not intellectualize what I am saying. It is your responsibility to experience your body and its state of health. When you feel how your body works, then, and only then, can you attempt to change it.

When you are giving a massage, it is helpful to take the receiver through some of these exercises. Both the giver and the receiver should be aware of the principles of holistic massage and health. These exercises can also be used as focusing devices before giving the massage. The purpose of focusing exercises is to gather together and focus the conscious awareness of both giver and receiver on the present moment and the task at hand. (See Chapter 14, "Meditation/Focusing," and Chapter 15, "The Giver," for more about focusing.)

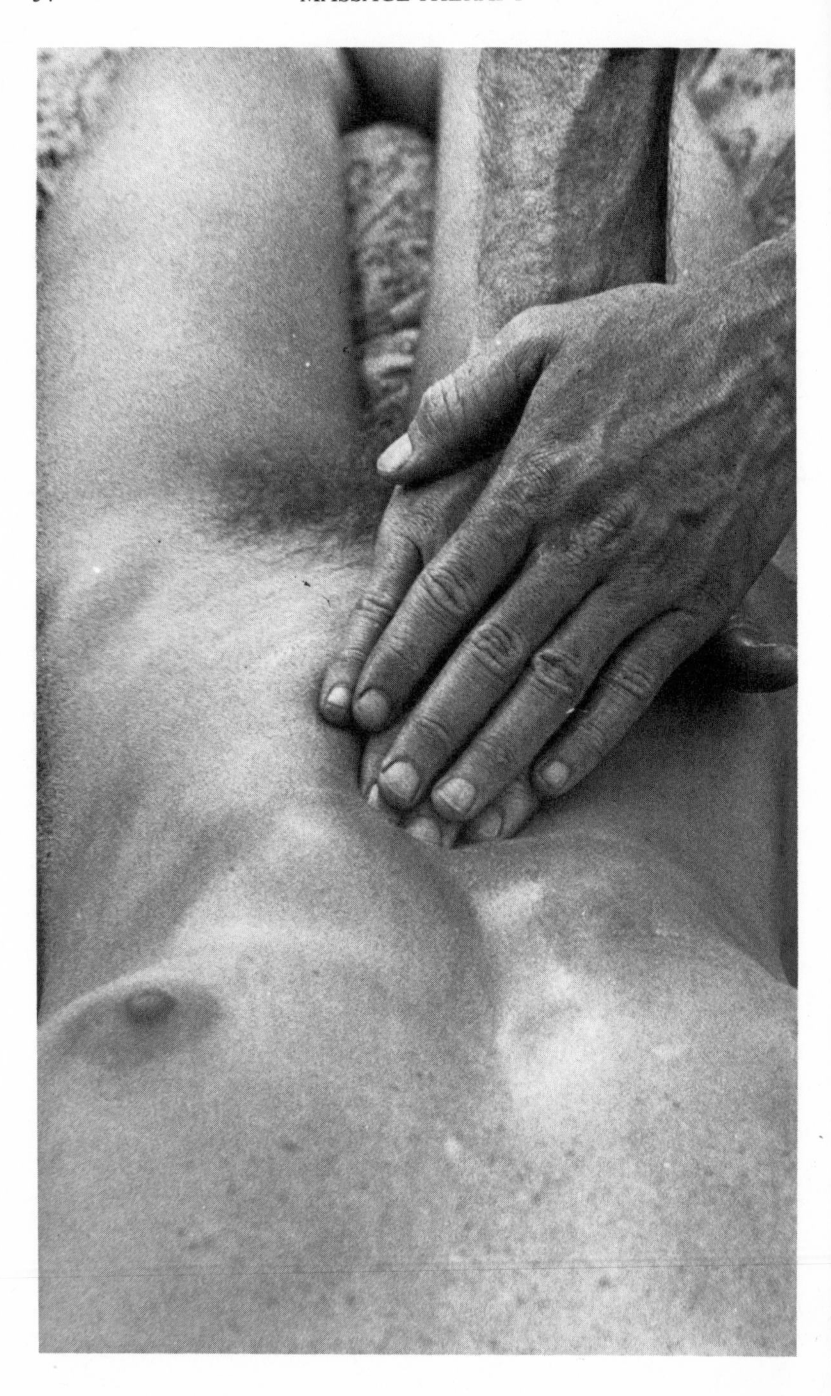

6.

Sickness as a Positive Life Force

Disease is an integral part of the human condition. There is no possible way we can eliminate it from our lives. Humankind evolves through health *and* sickness. We learn from both. We see sickness as bad, so we attack it through powerful, and often harmful, drugs. Pain is seen as something to be avoided at all costs. Any hint of discomfort calls for a pill or a visit to the doctor. Is it that we cannot cope as individuals with our own natural cycles of evolution? Most often doctors and drugs serve only to make illness less painful. The body has its own ways of coping with physical imbalance, and drugs often prolong or interfere with the body's natural healing processes. Modern medicine is preoccupied with ridding or masking symptoms, and this may be a major reason why it is so ineffective.

Each of us carries the potential to contract any disease at any time. However, only certain people actually do become ill, whereas others remain well. Although good diet and good health habits are important to staying healthy, they do not completely explain why only some people become sick and others do not. There *must* be something more to health than we have previously considered.

Medicine is at a crossroads today. The development of the fields of psychiatry, hypnosis, and holistic health, coupled with explorations into the nature of consciousness, give convincing evidence that we as individuals cause most, if not all, of our own health problems. Conservative estimates indicate that 75 percent of illnesses are psychosomatic, whereas more liberal estimates reach 95 percent. "Psychosomatic" does not mean that the illness does not exist in reality. It simply means that illness is caused by the action of the mind (psyche) on the body (soma). The illness is very real. As this view gains acceptance, it is changing our whole concept of the causes of illness. What we have previously considered as *causes* of illness now can be seen as only the *agents* of change. The real causes lie deeper than we ever considered.

Viewed holistically, the individual is seen as having conscious control over, and responsibility for, his own health. Why do we create sickness for ourselves, and what useful purpose could it serve?

If you carefully review your health and personal history, the answers to these questions may become clear. You may find that most of your health problems have served a useful purpose. Granted, the reason for a particular illness is not often apparent at the time, but things are most often clearer in retrospect. Often, illness serves more than one purpose. Sometimes illness is a built-in defense mechanism that helps you to avoid life situations that you just cannot face or to avoid doing things you do not want to do. Sociologists have observed that some people seem to choose sick roles in certain relationships or social settings.

Sometimes you may be working too hard and get yourself into a situation in which you need a break, but you cannot just take a day off. Possibly, at times, your answer to this type of dilemma has been to become sick. Or maybe there are times when you find life depressing and need more love, sympathy, or attention. An illness might very well fulfill your needs.

Often there is a lesson to be learned. The inner self (subconscious) demonstrates limitless power. This self appears to use sickness as a teaching tool for the conscious self. If you had conscious ego control over this mechanism, you probably would have avoided many of the more important lessons you have learned in life out of fear or misunderstanding. You may find that when you are not very empathetic to another person's life situation or when you are expressing yourself in ways that are contrary to your natural energy flows, sickness often teaches you to be less cruel or selfish and more understanding. If you relate to yourself and all of life's creations with respect and love, you will find that all aspects of health—physical, mental, and spiritual—improve.

Besides learning individual lessons, we can benefit from group lessons as well. Life is precious and must not be violated through gross pollution. In the past twenty years, we have polluted our air, water, land, and food. The incidence of cancer in the United States is reaching epidemic proportions, and it is estimated that most cancers are environmentally caused. But we cannot treat cancer, a symptom of human decay, without recognizing and eliminating its cause—not the pollution itself, but our attitudes toward life that created the pollution. Pollution is not the cause of cancer; it is only the *agent* of change. Individual health and group health are questions of balance.

To view sickness as a positive life force is to accept the belief that the body is more than a mechanical entity. It is something more than a physical organism reacting to and adapting to its environment. There are mental and spiritual aspects that are integral to the state of health of the physical being.

The physical body is an outward expression of the inner self. It reflects the inner condition through thoughts, feelings, ideas, and emotions—not only about ourselves but also about others and about life in general. The inner self (subconscious) attempts to communicate to the conscious self through health, sickness, pain, and so on. This holistic view makes self-awareness of primary importance in achieving and maintaining optimal health. An individual must be honestly aware of his inner condition before the physical condition can be constructively and permanently changed.

I am not trying to tell you why you get sick, and I am not trying to tell you how to eliminate sickness from your lives. Such a thing would be impossible, because sickness is an integral part of the human condition. My purpose is to make you aware of aspects of health that you may not have considered before. The real reasons for sickness involve more than germs or infections alone. It is important to keep in mind that sickness is ultimately a positive life force. Sickness can both teach an individual and help him to fulfill a variety of needs. Avoid judging sickness or people who are sick. There is nothing to be judgmental about. It is a natural learning process. Try not to fall into the trap of dwelling on symptoms or despairing about your condition or self-image. Health is a dynamic process. If you are sick, begin by honestly searching within yourself for the *real* causes of the illness. Replace negative thoughts and feelings with positive ones and try to be honest with yourself and others. Relate to yourself and all of life with respect and love. Sickness is not a sign of weakness. Rather, it is a signal for growth.

Seen in this way, sickness is a positive life force to be used constructively as a learning process. This can also make sickness more bearable. We can have confidence that there is a good reason for illness, and we can realize that we are not just being knocked around by the currents of life. We, as individuals, are in control of our health.

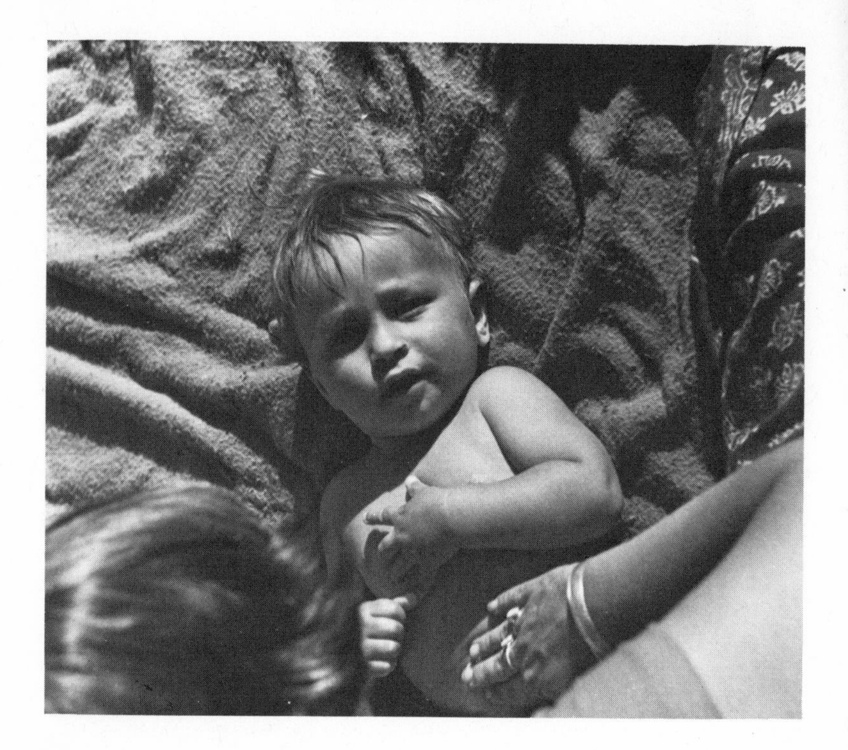

7.

Effects of Holistic Massage

The three components of body/mind/spirit are inseparable. Anything that affects one aspect will have an effect on the others. Many effects of massage are obvious and have been extensively studied, whereas others are more subtle and are limited only by our ability to perceive them.

Each massage is individual. There will be different effects produced, depending on the particular massage or technique used. In this chapter, I will elaborate on some of the effects of holistic massage. Use your own experience to add to the list. Massage affects us similarly in many ways and differently in others, and I do not presume to have experienced all of the benefits that massage has to offer.

The Giver

Whenever discussing the effects of massage, most books concentrate on the physiological effects on the receiver. During holistic massage, however, the giver can receive many very positive psychological benefits. It might be helpful to list a few possibilities here and allow you to add to the list as you experience them through practice.

The giver of a holistic massage is most effective when he develops an intimate feel for the muscles and other tissues. He should try to work the soft tissues gently, with a close, inner sense of what is being done and of how he wants the tissues to respond. It is necessary for the giver to try to develop an inner contact and rapport with the muscles. In so doing, he can blend with the receiver and become more effective in influencing the condition of the muscles.

When touching someone, it should be with the intent of making that person feel better. During holistic massage the giver will sense a rhythm, harmony, and flow developing as a result. This can be a source of pleasure, delight, and self-satisfaction. Holistic massage can arouse feelings of joy, peace, and contentment within the giver, both through the process of giving the massage and from the results experienced by the receiver.

Holistic massage is a good way to get to know someone and to develop a close relationship based on honesty and trust. This happens because of the very nature of the experience. Holistic massage brings two people together to work toward a positive benefit to the health of both participants. I honestly feel this is a very high order of communication. There is no room for the many psychological games people play. Holistic massage can affect relationships in many positive ways. Anything that decreases feelings of isolation and opens communication between two people is healthy for both.

Other effects of giving a massage include the satisfying and rewarding feelings you will receive from working with people and the high-energy experience that usually develops during and after a massage. These are some of the effects holistic massage can have on the giver. When he is able to blend into the flow of the experience, it is a very refreshing, exhilarating, and healthy event. All of these effects depend on a number of variables related to the psychological attitudes of the giver before and during a massage. The giver can have a completely miserable time if he does not feel like giving a massage and ends up giving one anyway.

The Receiver

The effects of massage on the receiver are probably even more numerous and include physiological as well as psychological results. The sensual joys are just as intense, probably even more so. When I receive a massage, the sensory input awakens long-lost areas of my body. The effects on body awareness are so numerous that they are dealt with in a separate chapter—Chapter 5. These sensual pleasures give me a peaceful, relaxed sense of well-being. I feel the caring touch of another, and it gives me a feeling of joy to know that someone cares enough to want to help me feel better.

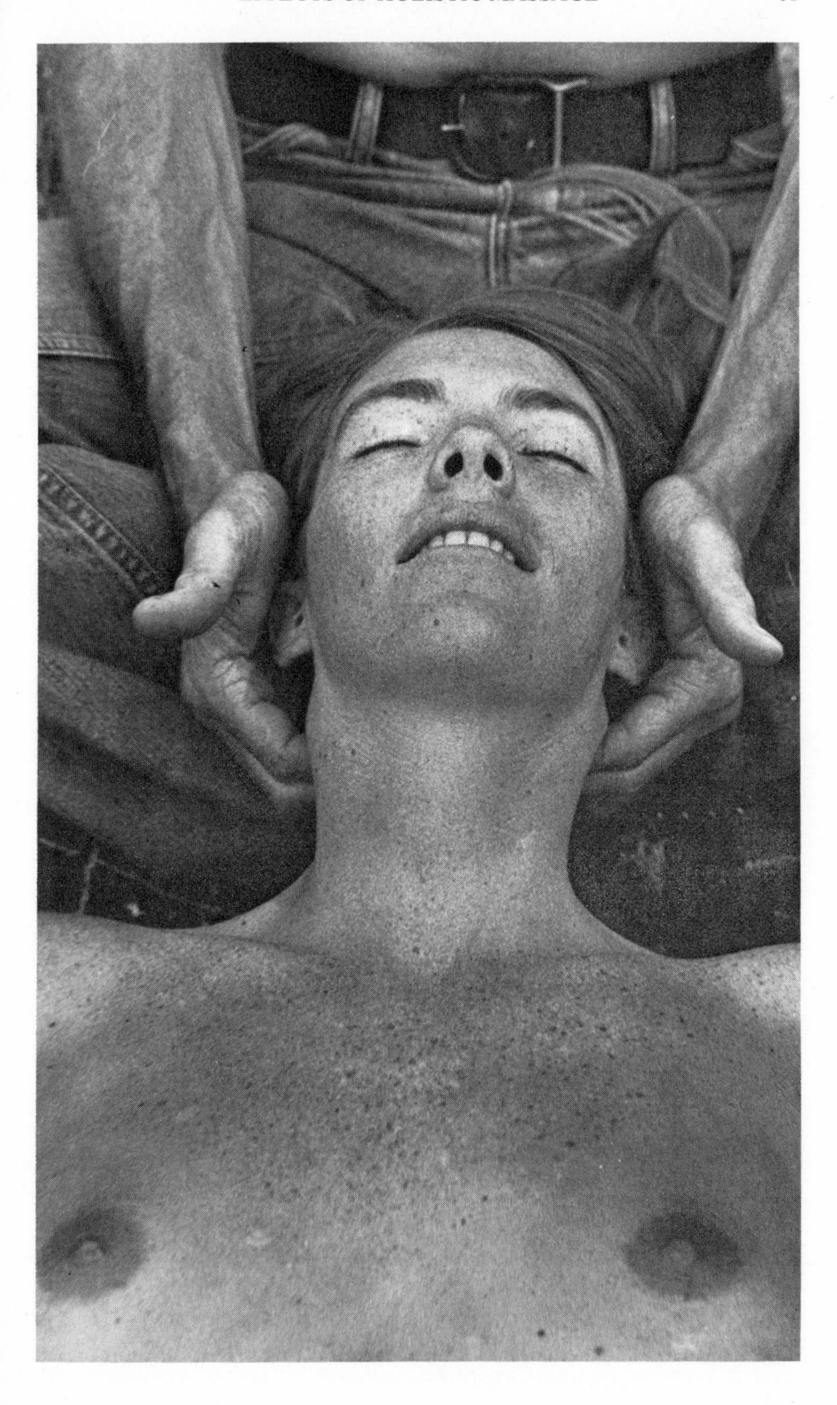

These benefits affect one's psychological well-being and develop sensations that have considerable healing benefits for the body and spirit alike.

Massage is also helpful in reducing painful tension and muscle spasms that result from injury or years of stored emotions. The sedative effects of massage cause a reflex reaction of the nerves that decreases muscle tension. This sedative effect on the nerves may also account for the decrease in pain impulses carried by the nerves to the brain.

One of the important effects of massage is the release of emotions and buried feelings as the tense muscles relax. The giver should be aware of this possibility and should actually encourage it. As tension caused by stored emotions is released through manipulation, the emotions are often unpleasant to realize and the receiver is often reluctant to expose his deepest emotions to another. Such emotional release is sometimes accompanied by tears. Clinical observation leads me to conclude that emotional release is a necessary part of therapy if long-term physical improvement is desired. I have seen people reach a plateau of physical improvement during long-term therapy and then go beyond that plateau when they finally deal with deep-seated emotional feelings. Often these feelings are accompanied by vivid images from the past that are associated with emotions. Sometimes there is a deep emotional release of tears that comes and goes without warning. Such events *always* produce positive physical and psychological changes. Areas of stubborn tension finally release, and the receiver feels good inside.

Emotional release can occur hours after a massage has ended, and the receiver should be prepared for this possibility. I have had people report that feelings of uneasiness have stayed with them for hours after a massage. These experiences seem to signal emotions that are refusing to be buried again until they are resolved. I encourage people to follow and explore their emotions and subjective feelings during and after the massage experience. When they do this, instead of ignoring their feelings, the emotions will pass by like free-flowing rivers. The receiver gains a greater insight into the cause of a particular pain or area of muscle tension. And the cause must be dealt with before lasting change can take place. The receiver is left with contentment through inner awareness instead of muscle tension and uneasiness.

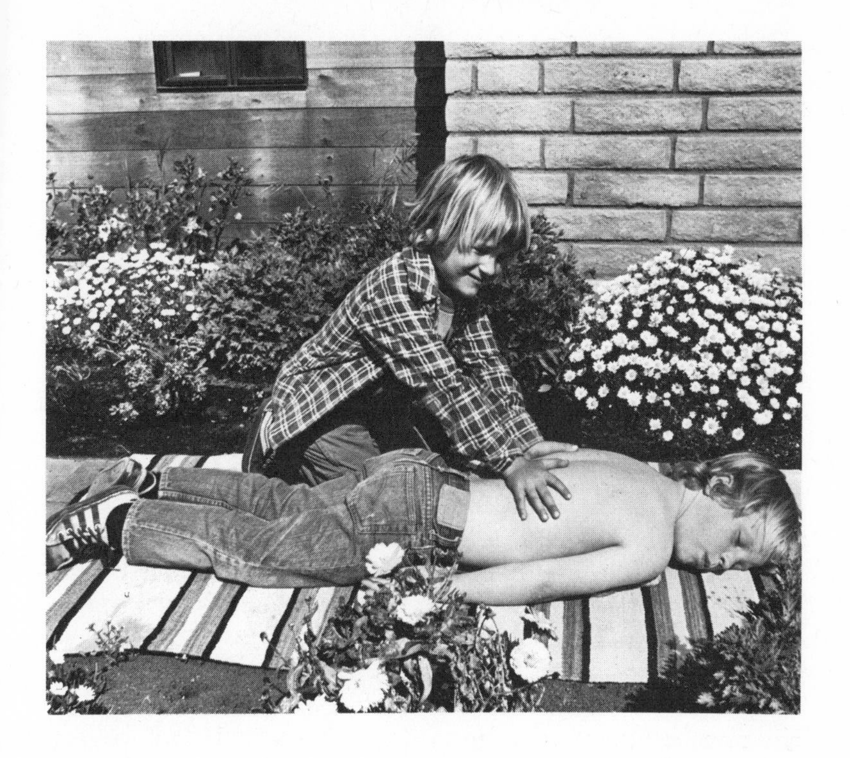

The giver should be aware that the receiver will only open up to someone he trusts. The giver must be worthy of this confidence by keeping what happens during a massage between the two people involved. The giver has to be sensitive to the privacy of the receiver.

Another benefit of holistic massage on the receiver are improvements in posture that result from the release of muscle tension. I mentioned before that muscle tension pulls the body out of its natural alignment. The stored emotions, expressed through muscle tension, also adversely affect posture. Our bodies reflect emotional attitudes. If we feel oppressed, we usually have a head-down, slouched posture. Other emotional attitudes produce their own characteristic postures. When emotions and muscle tensions are released, there is a corresponding improvement in posture. These effects are gradual and can be best viewed during long-term therapy, when people report feelings of lightness, ease of motion, and an increased feeling of natural energy flow.

It has been demonstrated experimentally that both superficial and deep stroking increase blood circulation as well as the amount of hemoglobin in the blood. Oxygen is carried throughout the body by hemoglobin; therefore, massage can increase the oxygen-carrying capacity of the blood. Body functions rely on oxygen. Injured tissues must have oxygen to rebuild themselves. It follows, then, that massage aids in the upkeep of the tissues and helps to remove the waste materials produced during injury, inflammation, and fatigue. The mechanical actions of the hands during a massage aid in returning blood to the venous system through which it is cleaned, oxygenated, and returned to the peripheries to aid in the healing process.

Increased circulation produces an environment within the tissues that is conducive to healing. A painful area is slow to heal because muscle spasms actually inhibit circulation. Muscles become sore partly because of a build-up of waste products from these constant contractions. One such product is lactic acid, which can only be metabolized in the presence of oxygen. Soreness sometimes persists after a massage because it takes time for the relaxed muscles to heal. Massage allows the healing process to begin. Massage in itself does not heal. It merely creates the conditions necessary for healing.

Many of the physical effects of massage occur as a result of the reflex activity of the autonomic (involuntary) nervous system. This system usually works reflexively, beyond our control. During massage, the general level of nervous tension is reduced, causing reduced muscle tension, increased circulation, and decreased heart rate and blood pressure and promoting a feeling of relaxation and well-being. These results not only heal the body but soothe the mind and strengthen the spirit. The simple act of relaxation causes a chain reaction of positive benefits within the body.

Giver and Receiver

A significant effect of holistic massage is that it promotes a feeling of well-being for both giver and receiver. It feels *so* good in *so* many ways. And anything that gives us a true feeling of inner happiness and well-being is beneficial to our health.

The giver and receiver also benefit spiritually from massage. Buddhists believe that one of the highest attainable spiritual states is the union of two people without sexual intercourse. I believe a similar union can happen during holistic massage when each partner's attention is focused and each is completely aware. The expanding of consciousness, the flight of intellect and ego, and the disappearance of time during massage all enhance spiritual awareness. This in turn acts to heal the body and the mind and to take us just that much closer to becoming complete and satisfied human beings. (See "Meditation/Focusing," Chapter 14.)

Viewed holistically, health is seen as a balance of mind, body, and spirit. Techniques that benefit the mind and spirit will in turn have positive and lasting effects on the body.

These results and more occur when massage is systematically applied in the manner I have described. If applied haphazardly, without thought or concern for the basic components of rate, rhythm, pressure, and direction, these results cannot be expected. The quality of the art is directly dependent upon the quality of the artist.

These effects happen to one degree or another during a single session. The body often suffers from years of misuse, tension, and anxiety. It is best to view massage as a dynamic process to be continued regularly throughout life. If you try for complete, permanent results in one massage, you will be discouraged. If you find muscle spasm and try to eliminate it completely in too short a time, you will become frustrated, as will the person receiving the mas-

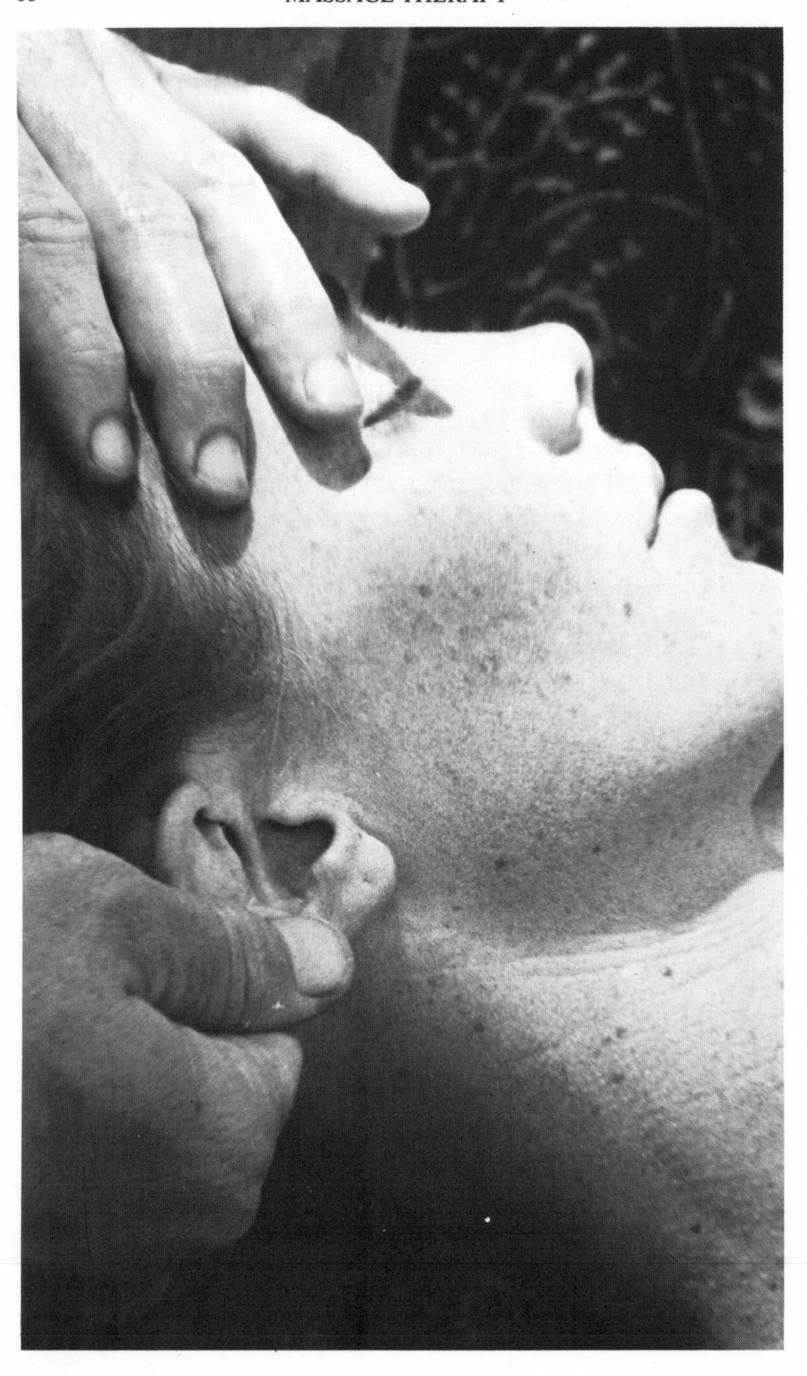

sage. It takes years to develop the muscle spasms we carry around. It is naive to think that they can be eliminated in one or two massage sessions. *Massage is a process.* Approach it as such, and results will follow at their own speed.

A Word of Caution

Massage is used to treat or aid in the treatment of a wide variety of physical problems. In fact, even if a massage has no significant physiological effect on a particular condition, it will usually have a positive psychological effect. There are a few conditions, though, that make massage dangerous. Massage should not be used to treat venous problems, such as thrombosis, acute phlebitis, or severe varicose veins. Acute inflammatory conditions (as occur in the presence of acute infection or for twenty-four hours after a severe sprain) may only be worsened by massage. In the case of musculoskeletal trauma (strains, sprains, and so on), cold applications are best initially, and after about one day massage can be of benefit. Skin conditions do not generally respond to massage and may even be spread further by massage. Too, acute systemic diseases, gastric or duodenal ulcers, and debilitating diseases in which complete bed rest is indicated may all be worsened with massage. Finally, massage should not be employed in the presence of large hernias, advanced arteriosclerosis, abscesses, aneurisms, or burns.

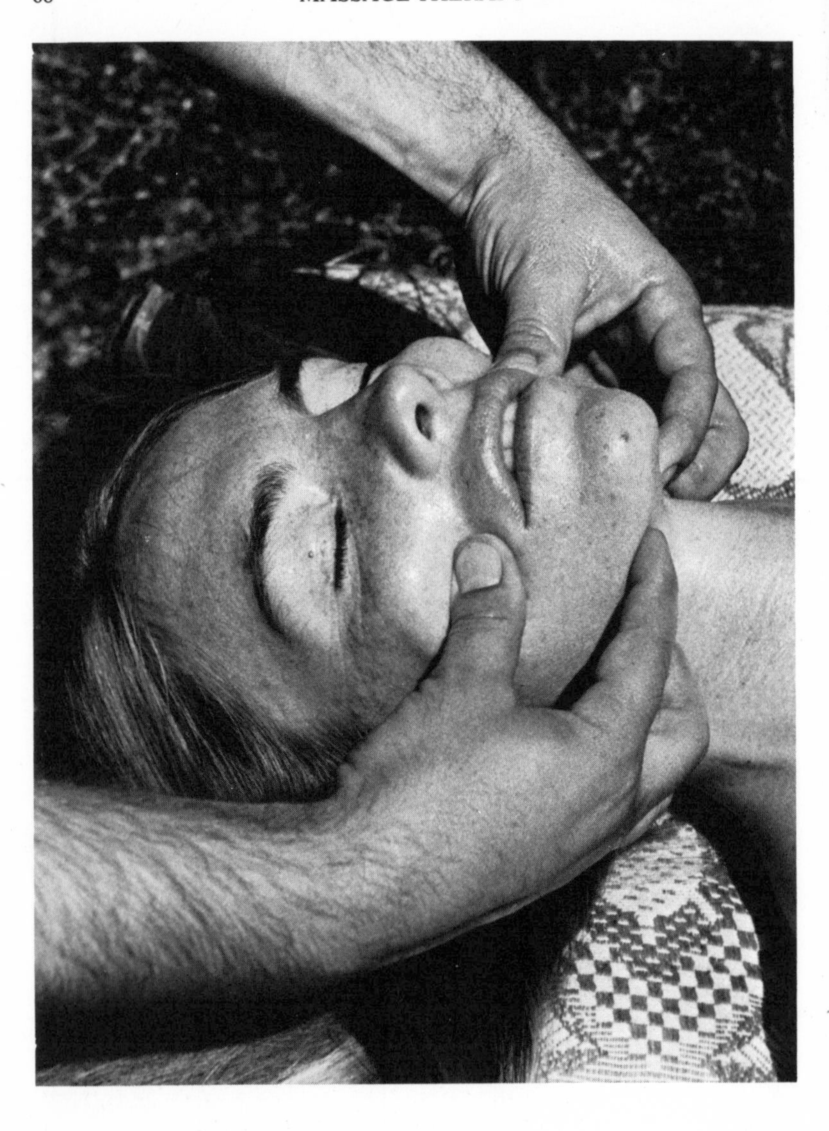

8.

Healers or Helpers?

You would not be reading this book if you did not want to help people feel better. Massage is a very direct and natural way to accomplish this. All of us have experienced seeing friends or loved ones sick and wanting to help them, or heal them, or somehow make them more comfortable.

I have mentioned our present dependency on doctors. We really expect them to heal us. Many of you may even wish to become healers. These concepts fit poorly in the holistic view of health, because they are based on the premise that some people have the power to heal others. Looking back on the people whom I have treated, it is not difficult to realize that individuals heal themselves. Rather than healing them, I have simply been an agent of change. This is not to negate the role of an agent. Helping others is a rewarding experience, but I try to keep my role in proper perspective, and I encourage you to do the same.

As you become more involved with massage and work with other people, you will find them eager to pass their responsibilities along to you. They will ask you to take away their problems. Be aware of this possibility and direct the responsibility back to them through holistic massage. We are helpers, *not* healers.

If you are working with another person and he fails to improve, do not despair. The responsibility and the credit for change, or the lack of it, rests ultimately with the patient. This is not to say that people cannot believe strongly in a healer's abilities and through that belief heal themselves. If you really want to help someone improve, give him self-confidence and reinforce the belief that he will improve. A person's condition cannot possibly improve until he first has the desire to change and the belief that his condition *will* improve. Your own attitudes and empathy for another's condition will help greatly in this area. You are a catalyst for change, and this is often all that is needed to effect that change.

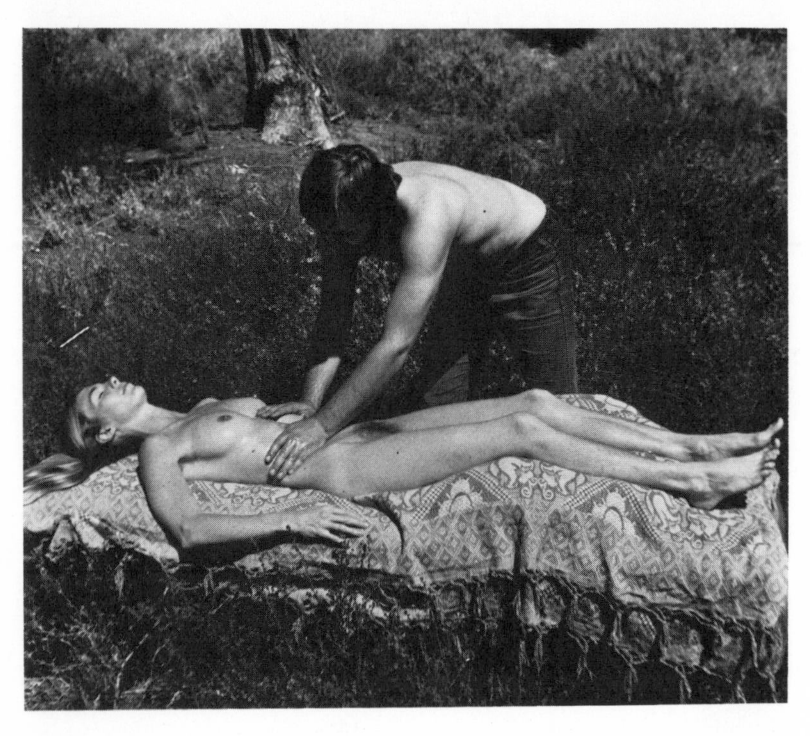

9.

Anatomy

A good massage is one in which the giver has a sense of direction and purpose during the experience. When the giver has confidence and direction, it is felt by the receiver. I have given you many clues to help you understand the basic components of massage and some areas of potential experience. Your understanding will not be complete until you have learned some basic anatomy. I believe a basic knowledge of what is under the skin is essential to giving a quality massage. When a person who is not at all familiar with anatomy gives a massage, something is always lacking.

Although human anatomy may appear confusing, I assure you it is not. Still, many people resist learning some fundamental, yet vital, information about the subject. I have seen the quality of a massage improve when a student finally lets down his defenses and spends an hour or so looking at muscle charts. The change is truly dramatic. The missing dimension of direction and purpose is gained.

Learning the names of the muscles does help in communicating to another person who is also familiar with the names, but that is about all it does. For this reason, I have refrained from extensively labeling the anatomy charts. What is more important is to get a picture of what structures lie under the skin and, in the case of muscles, which way their fibers run. That is basically all you really have to know, and I assure you it is not complicated.

Massage is an excellent way to become familiar with the human body's tensions, strengths, and weaknesses. Not many people are aware of what lies under their skin, and massage helps both giver and receiver become more aware of how the human body is built.

With an understanding of body structure and function, it is possible to understand everyday aches and pains a little better. Working on the body without knowing its component parts and their locations is like trying to fix a car engine without knowing anything about mechanics. The process of working on something, whether a body or a car, with an honest desire to learn how it operates, can be a richly rewarding experience. It becomes obvious when working on complicated machinery that, in the beginning, the work may entail considerable probing and exploration. Maybe you will need an instruction manual or schematic diagram. Gradually, however, you develop an understanding of how the machine works. You begin to get a feel for what is wrong and what is functioning properly, and your attempts at repair take on direction and purpose. This same process will occur when you are learning massage. At first, when someone comes to you with a specific complaint, you will be poking and probing without much idea of what you are doing. But gradually you will begin to see and feel how certain complaints relate to certain muscles. Much like a car with a bad fuel pump that creates specific symptoms, a bad muscle exhibits identifiable indications of specific problems.

Injury is *always* accompanied by muscle spasm. Refer to Figures 3 and 4 to help you get an idea of how a muscle contracts and what a muscle spasm really is. Muscles are made up of fibers that run parallel to each other. Fibers are grouped together to form bundles, and bundles are grouped together to form a muscle belly. Muscles are often compared to wires in a telephone cable to illustrate how they are put together. When a muscle contracts, the individual fibers shorten. Each fiber is made up of filaments that interlock, much like your fingers interlock when you clasp your hands together. Physiologists believe that muscles contract when a nervous impulse stimulates the muscle, causing the filaments to slide over one another. This can be easily demonstrated when you interlock your fingers. As in your fingers, there are degrees of muscle contraction. Some contractions are transient, and other contractions are static. This static contraction is called "tetanic." Muscle spasm is a tetanic contraction in which a few or all of the fibers of a muscle are contracted to their maximum. A tetanic contraction occurs in one of two ways. One way is a reflex response to injury. Pain causes spasm, causing more pain, which in turn causes more spasm. The other way a muscle can go into tetanus is via long-term emotional tension. I have described how emotion causes us to tense our muscles. This tension is initially a mild contraction. An example is the tension experienced when driving in heavy traffic. As tension builds, the driver's shoulders gradually rise. Prolonged emotional stress causes muscles to contract maximally, and this condition, sometimes prolonged for a number of years, results in chronic, tetanic contraction. This is commonly called nervous tension, and it is a prime cause of physical disability. It distorts our bodies, causing postural imbalances, and is a major cause of headaches and chronic back pain.

Muscle spasm presents itself as a firm, hard lump of tissue. Sometimes, because of the firmness of these spasms, it is difficult to distinguish them from bones. This is another good reason to learn some basics of anatomy. The more practice you have giving massages, the easier it will be for you to identify muscle spasm. It is a sense that comes only with practice. Spasm can be as small as a pea or as large as a golf ball. In the case of the long back muscles, the spasm sometimes feels like a long, thin roll of hard rubber running under the skin and parallel to the spine.

To get an idea of what a spasm feels like, feel the middle of the triangular trapezius muscles of the shoulders (see Figure 6). It is very rare not to find some degree of spasm there. Spasm is best located by running the ball of your thumb over the length of a muscle, following the grain of the fibers. Again, knowing some anatomy is helpful in determining in which direction the fibers run for any particular muscle. As your thumb passes over the spasm, you will feel it as a definite lump or change in the tension of the muscle belly. Normal muscle tissue should be soft and pliable. Muscle tension is common all along the base of the skull, in the middle of the upper trapezius, along the borders of the scapula, and throughout the deep muscles that run adjacent to the spine (refer to Figure 7 for a look at the deep muscles). As you become adept at locating muscle spasm, you will find that these are the major problem areas.

Occasionally you will find a person who is quite hard throughout his body. Usually, this is the result of long-standing, low-grade body tension. Generally, when muscles are tense for a long time, inner structural changes occur. The muscles are infiltrated with connective tissue, the fibrous tissue that holds our bodies together. As a result, muscles tend to become hard, and the *only* thing that can free muscles of this tension is regularly scheduled massage. It takes years to develop this condition, and it will take a considerable amount of concentrated therapy to facilitate normal muscle tone. If you run across someone with hard muscles or if you have them yourself, do not despair. It is a common condition often caused by

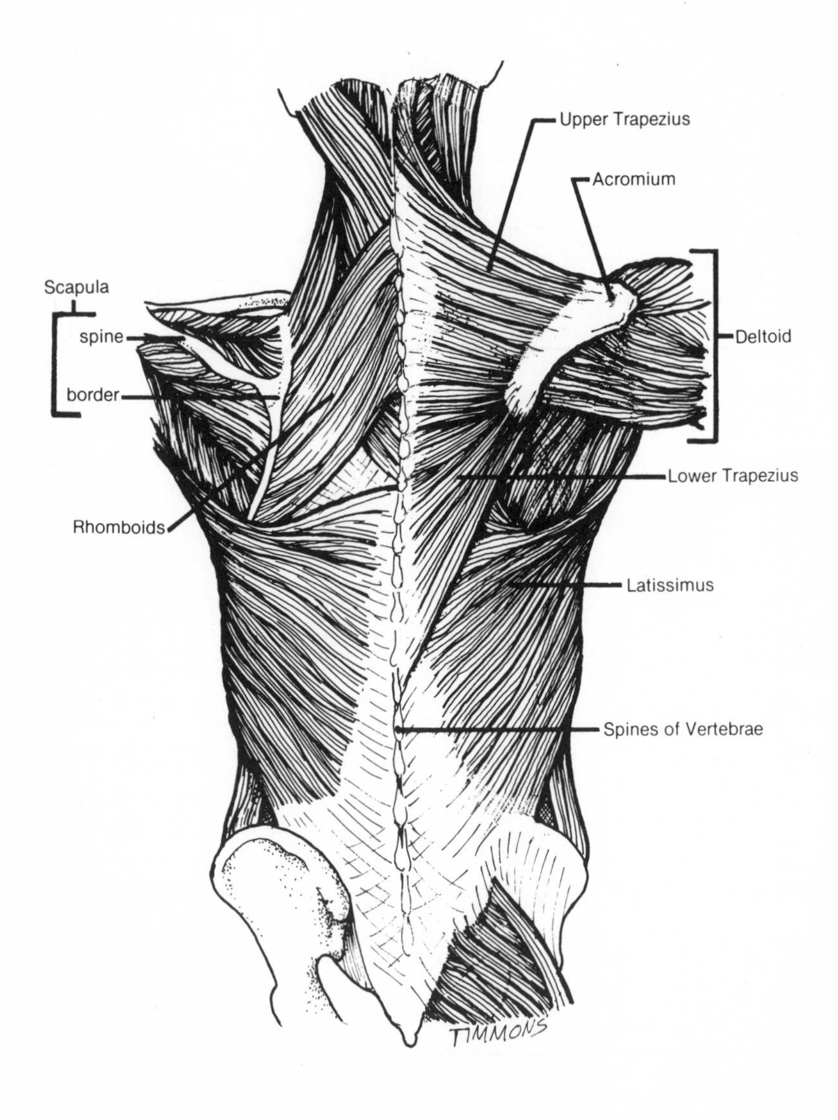

Figure 6. **The Full Back.** Notice that the trapezius and the deltoid have been removed on the left side to expose the underlying structures. The labeled structures are easily felt during a massage.

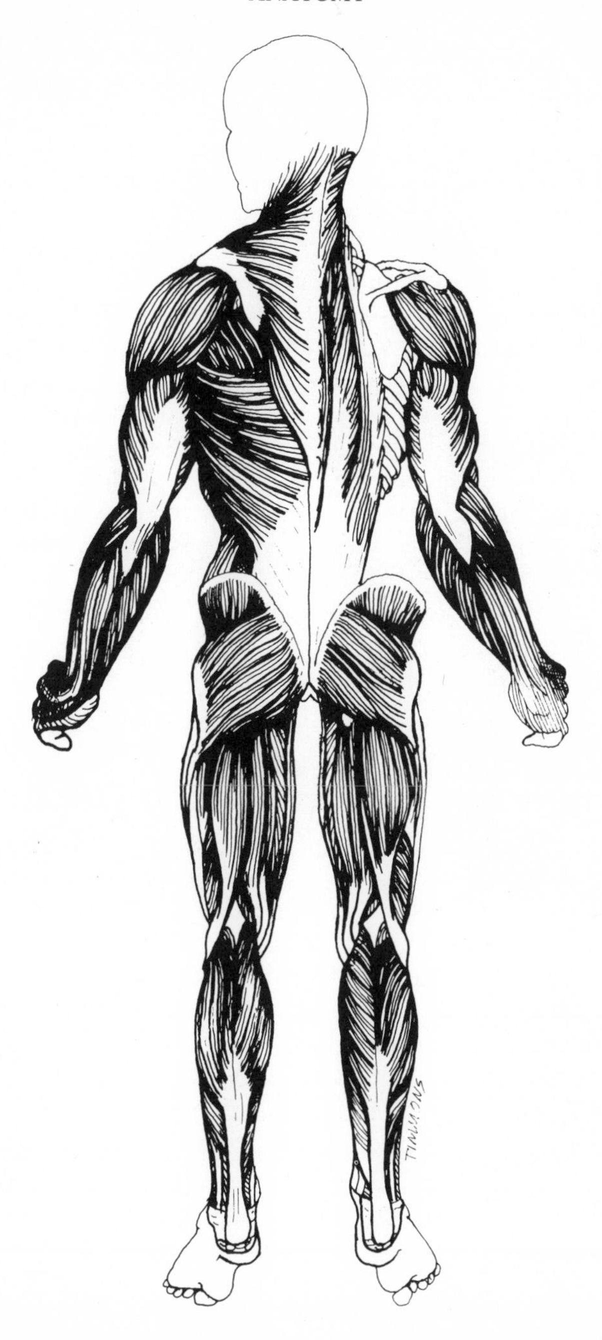

Figure 7. **The Full Body – Back View.** Notice that the deep muscles along the right side of the spine have been exposed. This area is often a source of tension and pain.

basic emotional attitudes. Our bodies shield themselves from the unknowns of life. Working with these people can be very rewarding because of the great deal of positive change you can effect through repeated massage. This is also a good situation in which to encourage emotional expression and inner exploration on the part of the receiver. People with full body muscle tension usually pride themselves on their invulnerability, so they are often hard to reach. When you break through their defenses, only then can you really help them. Surprisingly enough, I cannot recall one case in which I have seen a woman who had really hard, fibrous muscles.

After you locate a lump or spasm, identify the muscle or muscles involved. Spasm may be felt as a localized lump, but the whole muscle will be affected. Therefore, while massaging, you must give special attention in the form of stroking or kneading to the entire length of the muscle. This is impossible if you do not know some muscle anatomy. The best way to reduce spasm is by stroking the length of the muscle in the direction that the fibers run. Think back to the sliding filament theory. It would not make sense to massage against the muscle fiber grain. Too, a muscle under chronic tension is often in spasm at the points where the muscle attaches to the bone. It is helpful to apply kneading actions or friction to these areas.

Another method that is helpful in reducing muscle spasm is to apply constant pressure directly over the spasm. Be sure to do this within the pain tolerance of the person receiving the massage. Just press on the muscle, using the ball of your thumb, and hold for about thirty seconds. Bear in mind that no single session will eliminate tension. The use of pressure also helps the receiver to locate and become aware of the degree of tension he has.

Use the accompanying Figures 6–9 to help you learn muscle and bone anatomy. Go slowly and make the learning process enjoyable. Look for small hills and valleys on the body's surface to help you identify the locations of certain muscles. Use your sense of touch to help guide you. The more you touch, stroke, and knead the tissues of others, the more sensitive your hands will become.

Experience

You will need a friend as a model for this exercise. Refer to Figure 6, the diagram of the full back. A few of the more prominent structures are labeled in Figure 6, and these should be readily iden-

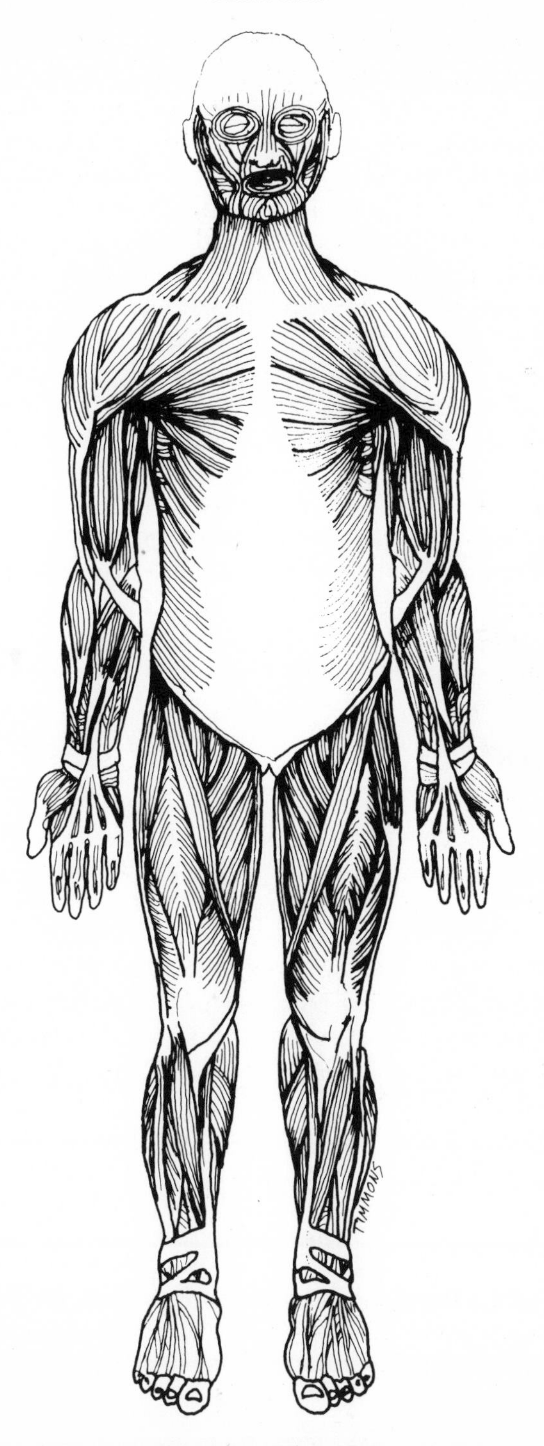

Figure 8. The Full Body – Front View.

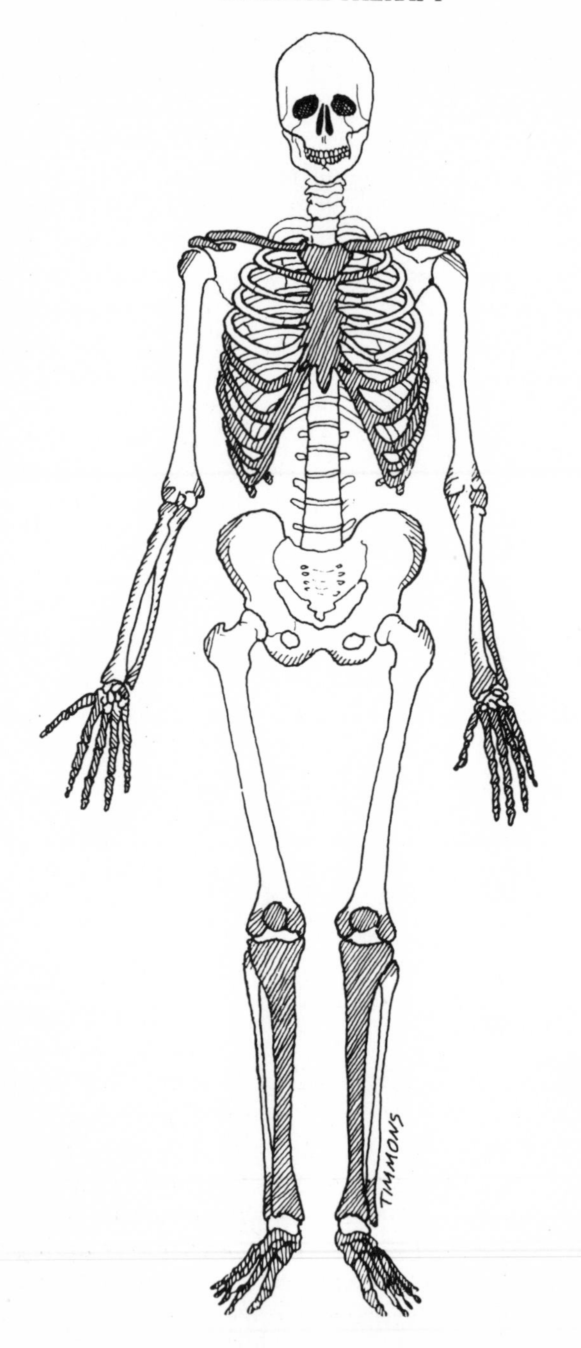

Figure 9. **The Human Skeleton.** The shaded areas are the bones that are close to the skin surface and felt during massage. Lighter pressure is always used over these areas.

tifiable by anyone interested in massage. First, try to palpate (feel with your fingertips) the spines of the vertebrae, from the top to the bottom of the spine. These are the points of bone that protrude toward the back. Next, locate the shoulder blade (scapula). You should be able to feel the spine of the scapula. This is a piece of bone that runs diagonally across the scapula and ends above the shoulder joint. At this point, it is called the acromium process. These two structures (scapular spine and acromium) are easily palpated and should not be mistaken for muscle spasm during a massage. Other structures that you can palpate are the borders of the scapula. Many muscles attach there, but the borders can be easily located.

Finally, identify the major muscles of the back. The large, triangular trapezius gives the sloping form to the upper shoulders, and the latissimus dorsi gives shape to the outside borders of the back.

Experience

Refer to Figure 9, the diagram of the skeleton. The bones, or parts of bones, that are close to the skin have been shaded. Using yourself as a model, try to palpate these structures. They are the areas where only light pressure is needed during massage.

If you combine this exercise with the previous one, you should not have difficulty distinguishing between muscles and bones during massage.

Experience

When you think you have sufficient anatomical knowledge, try testing yourself by using a concept like Braille. This is most rewarding with a loved one, so that your own inhibitions or those of the receiver will not interfere with the learning process. Have the receiver remove his clothes and lie down in a darkened room. When he is ready, massage his body without the benefit of sight. See how many muscles and other body structures you can locate by touch alone. Get into the habit of closing your eyes during massage. This has the effect of forcing you to focus completely on the receiver and on the massage experience as well.

PART II

THE BODY: MASSAGE TECHNIQUE

"See me . . .
Feel me . . .
Touch me . . .
Heal me . . ."
—From the rock opera *Tommy*

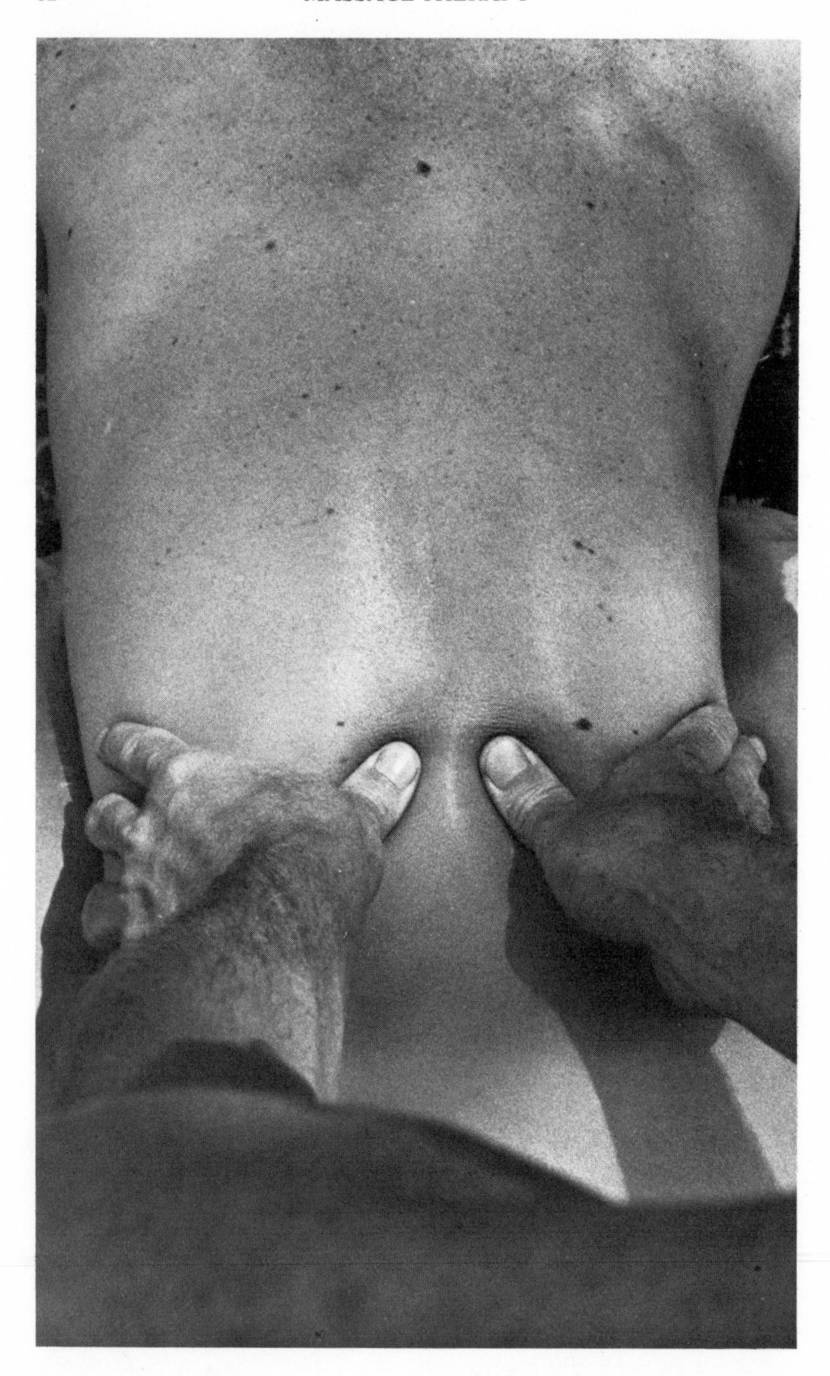

10.

Basic Components of Massage

Pressure

Every massage should begin with light stroking, and each subsequent stroke should be firmer than the one before. The transition from very light strokes to the very deepest ones should not be obvious to the receiver. The tissues of the body need to be warmed and coaxed into relaxation. Too rapid a progression to deeper strokes is both unnatural and uncomfortable. The receiver will react by tensing up rather than relaxing, thus defeating the purpose of massage. The first two thirds of a massage should be performed by increasing the pressure with each stroke. During the final portion, the pressure should be gradually decreased. (See Figure 10.)

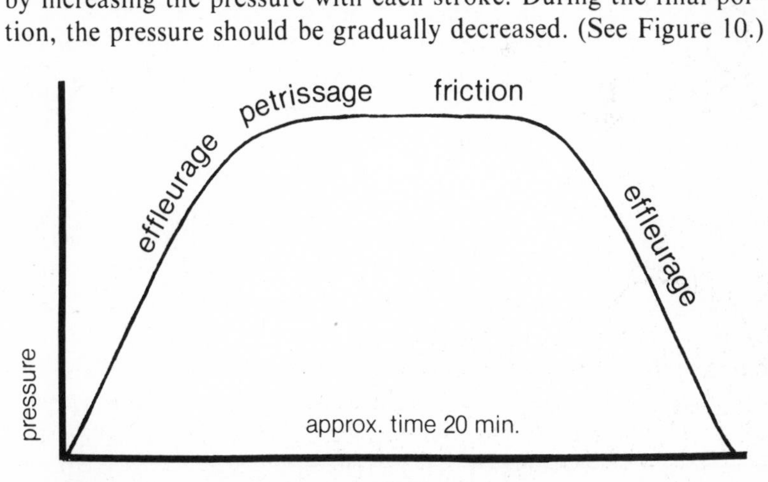

Figure 10. **Pressure Gradient.** During a massage, pressure should increase gradually, level off, and then gradually decrease.

Obviously, any abrupt change in pressure gradients will be felt by the receiver, and his body will react accordingly.

Pressure should be used on upward strokes, and return strokes should be light. Always attempt to push fluids toward the center or top of the body, rather than pushing out toward the periphery.

Speed

The rate with which you conduct the massage is critical in establishing rapport with your subject and in making him feel secure and confident with you. Massage is done in a slow, deliberate, and relaxed manner. If you hurry, your friend will feel it.

A rapid massage causes a person to become tense rather than relaxed, and this does not allow that inner flow of energies to develop between giver and receiver. If you do not have enough time to give a good massage, then do not give one at all.

The speed of a massage should be consistent throughout. If one part is a little faster than another, it breaks up the massage, creating a series of separate massages rather than a fluid, holistic experience.

Rhythm

Your whole body should experience the act of giving a massage. Strive to establish a rhythm in the way you move and breathe that remains consistent throughout the massage. Search for the natural rhythm, and giving a massage will not become a tiring experience. Review Chapter 2 for a more complete understanding of how breathing relates to movement.

I find it difficult to massage to music. The rhythm usually changes with each song and often changes within a single song. This creates conflicts and problems of energy flow for me. There are some types of music that are conducive to good massage, but I recommend you pick your music carefully. Actions in response to any factor other than the people involved in a massage often work against the experience. Massage requires total concentration on the experience and not on external happenings.

Rhythm will set the tone of the massage and will be useful in controlling your energy flow. If your movements and breathing are rhythmic, then the receiver's breath and consciousness will fall into that rhythm.

Position

It is important for both the giver and the receiver to be comfortable during the massage experience. The photographs in this book should give you a good idea of some possible positions from which to work. When the receiver is on his stomach, it is advisable to place a small pillow under the stomach to support the lower back, and it adds even more comfort to place a pillow under his shins. When the receiver is on his back, it may be more comfortable to place a pillow under his knees.

The most important thing to remember is always to move with your entire body, feeling the movement originate from your weight center, a point located two inches behind and below your navel. (See Chapter 14, "Meditation/Focusing.") If you massage with just your arms and hands, you will tire easily. It is also good practice to avoid overusing your back muscles. This is most important when massaging on the floor. Again if your forward and return movements originate from your center, your back will not be overworked. This applies to circular motions as well. Your whole body should be working. *Your hands are an extension of your entire body and its movements.*

If you must lean over from the side to reach the receiver, you will quickly become fatigued. When working on a table, have the receiver move as close to you as is comfortably possible. When working on the floor and applying long strokes from the side, it might be helpful to bend one leg to allow you to place your weight on the knee of the other leg. Experiment to find a position that is comfortable for you, and use it.

All massage should include the components I have described. At first you may have to remind yourself constantly of these things, but soon they will become habit. It cannot be overemphasized that both the giver *and* the receiver should be as comfortable as possible. This important aspect of position will facilitate the most rewarding massage experience.

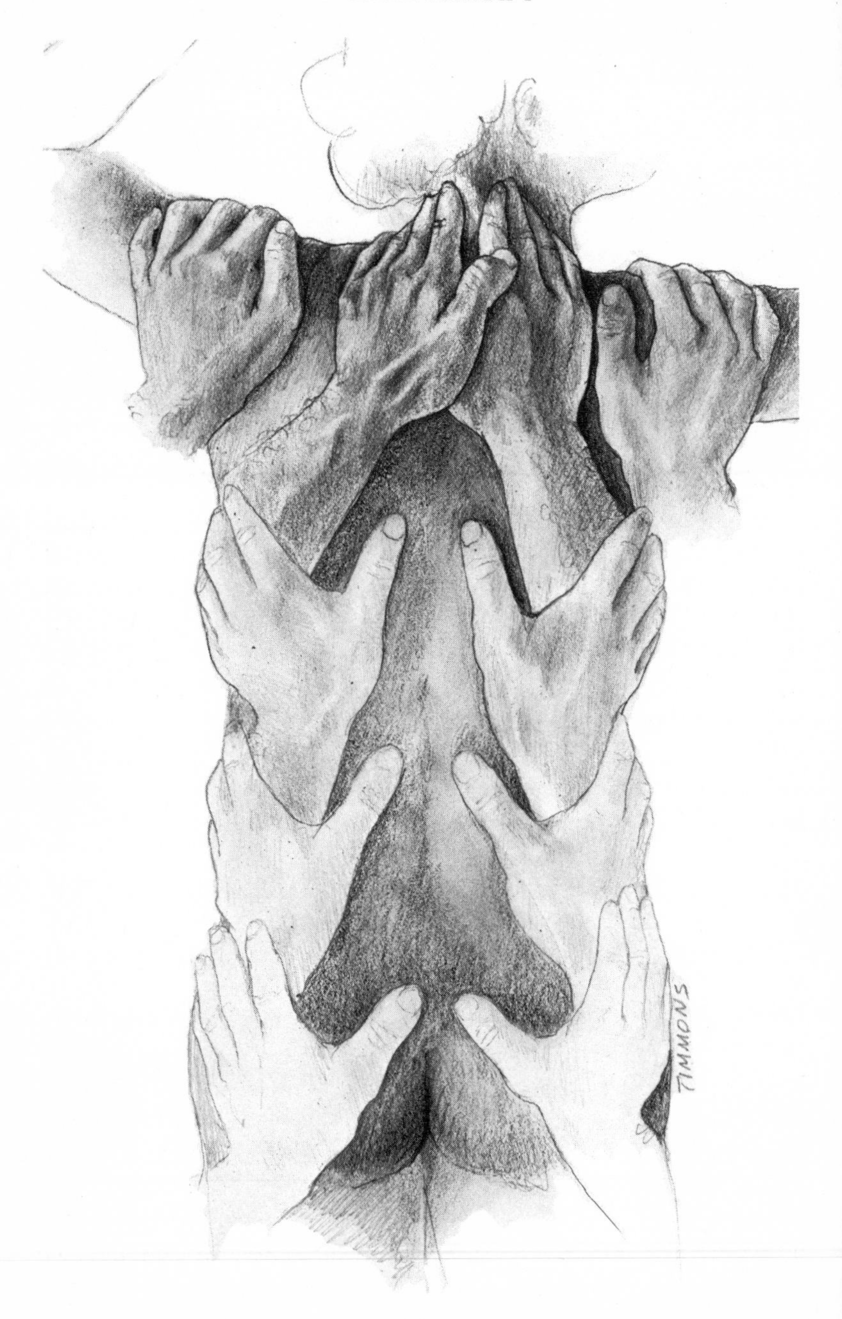

Figure 11. **Effleurage.** The hands begin at the buttocks and proceed smoothly to the neck.

11.

Basic Strokes

I have noticed that authors of massage books describe as many as eighty different massage strokes. This is one of the reasons I have written this book. *Massage has four basic strokes, and you should not have to learn more.*

1. *Effleurage (superficial stroking):* This is a longitudinal stroke of light to moderate pressure. Massage should always begin and eventually end with effleurage. This warms the tissues, allowing you to establish rhythm and flow, and helps you to get in touch with the body on which you are working. It also aids in calming the receiver. This stroke is usually executed on the full length of the back or other parts of the body (Figure 11).

2. *Petrissage (circular or deep transverse stroking):* This is a moderate to deep stroke, often circular or transverse in motion. During these deep motions you can feel the muscles and other tissues and discern in which areas the problems lie. Do not forget to perform petrissage with your whole body and not just with your arms and hands. I find it convenient to use two petrissage manipulations: two-handed circles and reinforced (hand-on-hand) circles (Figures 12 and 13).

Kneading is usually included as a petrissage movement, because it is a deep manipulation. However, because of its distinct character and use, I have listed it as a separate stroke.

3. *Kneading:* Kneading is executed on the underlying tissues by using the thumb and fingers of your hands, much as you would knead bread dough (Figure 14).

Kneading is a deep manipulation, done at will throughout the massage. This stroke is an important expressive and spontaneous manipulation and can be administered often. I usually perform kneading after petrissage and again after friction, concentrating my efforts on the problem areas I have found.

4. *Friction:* This describes deep, circular motions using the thumbs, knuckles, or ends of the fingers. Pressure is thereby con-

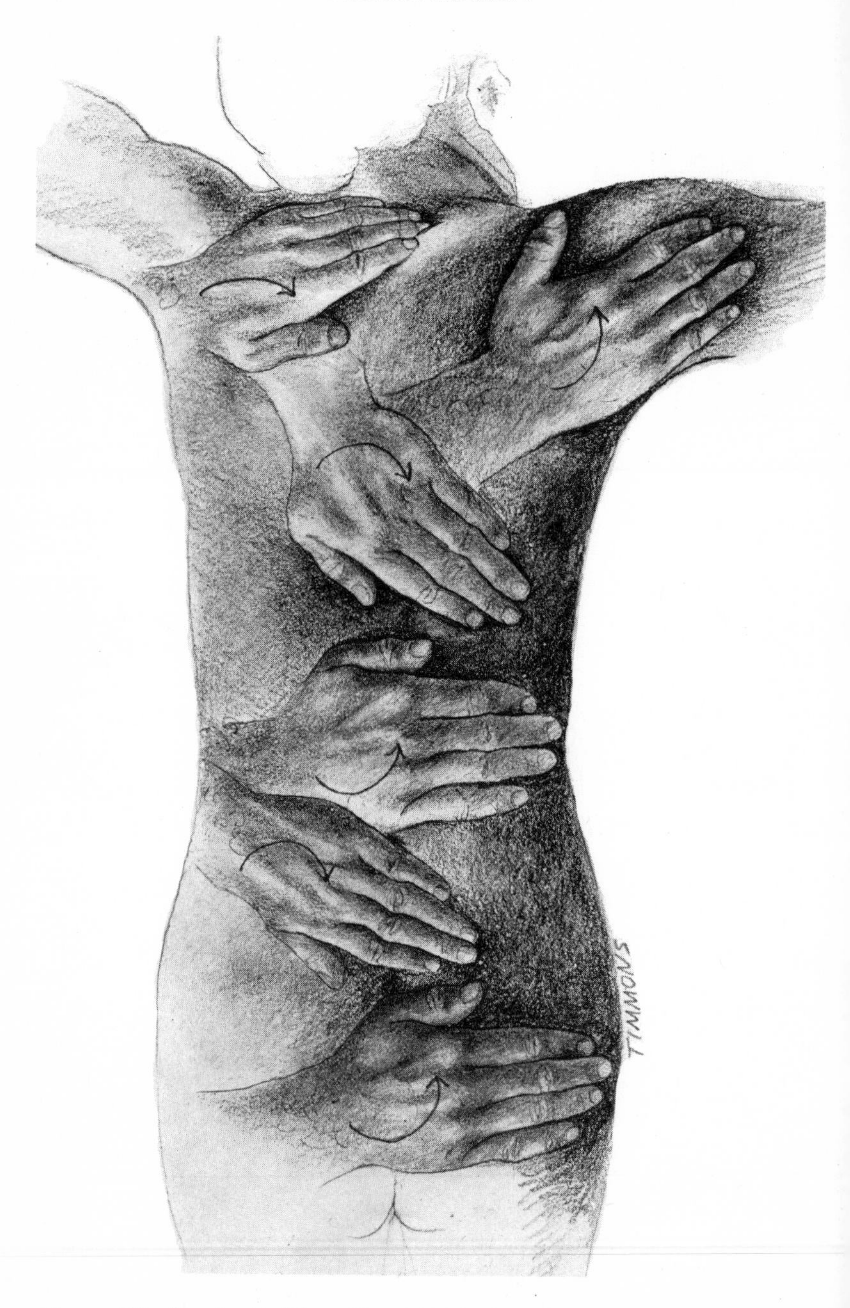

Figure 12. **Petrissage/Two-Handed Circles.** Starting at the buttocks, you proceed up the side. Notice that the right hand is moving in counterclockwise circles while the left is moving clockwise. When massaging the left side, the fingertips are adjacent to the spine.

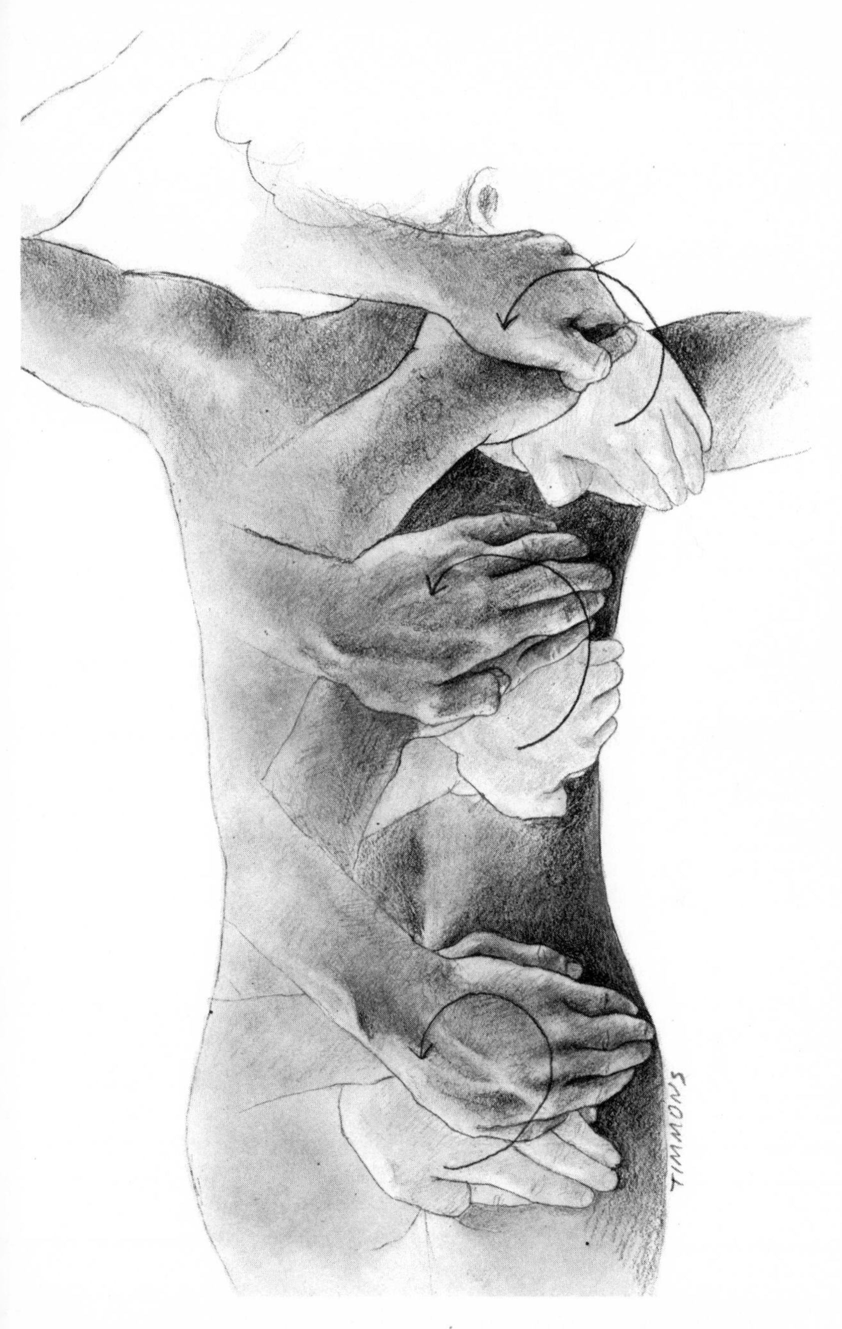

Figure 13. **Petrissage/Reinforced Circles.** Starting at the buttocks, the hands move in counterclockwise circles up the back. When switching to the left side, the hands should follow a clockwise pattern.

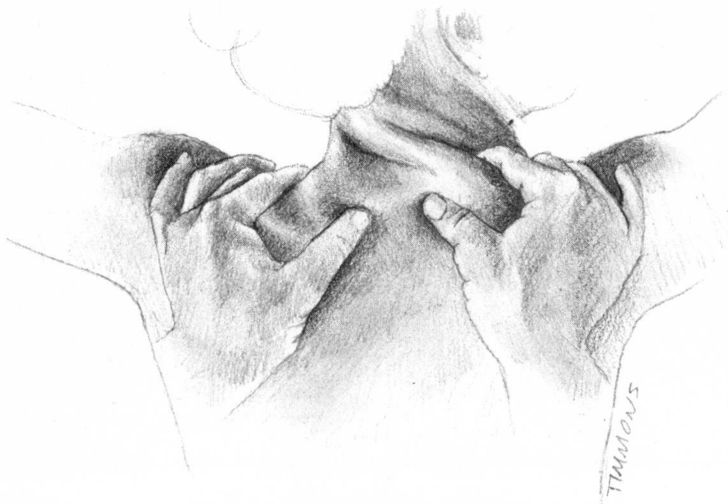

Figure 14. **Kneading.**

centrated in a small area. When working with your thumbs, use your hands for support. Make deep circles about the size of a half-dollar coin with your thumbs and *slowly* work your way up the spine (see Figure 15). Of course, friction can be used anywhere throughout the body. Friction is the deepest manipulation you can apply without causing pain.

I follow deep circular motions (petrissage) with friction along either side of the spine and then over problem areas as needed. In relation to the pressure gradient, friction is the deepest used and should remain within the limits of the receiver's comfort.

These are the basic strokes used in a massage intended to relax the muscles specifically and the body generally. The technique chapters that follow describe how to use these strokes during a massage. From there, your creativity can assume control. These four strokes form the basic skeleton of massage from which you can work. To become any more technical or involved would make massage too mechanical and rigid.

Classic Swedish massage employs some very vigorous strokes, which most people associate with massage. Swedish massage is designed to stimulate, not to relax. The strokes include slapping, percussion, and beating, among others. I feel that this type of massage is far too vigorous for most purposes. The receiver seems more intent on survival and on blocking body sensations than on relaxing and increasing body awareness. If your goal is to stimulate someone, then by all means use these manipulations. But do so within the tolerance level of the receiver.

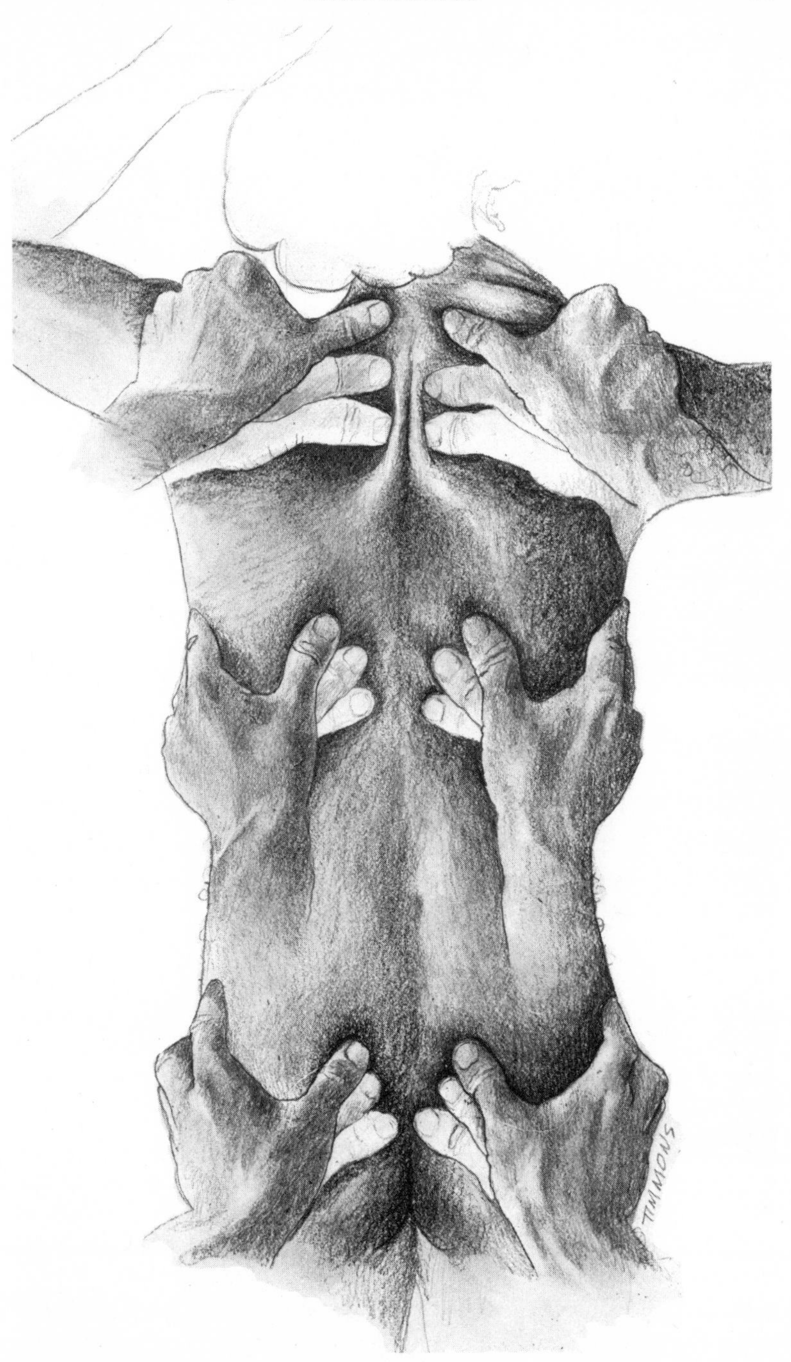

Figure 15. **Friction.** Starting at the base of the spine, the thumbs trace small circles and gradually work up the spine.

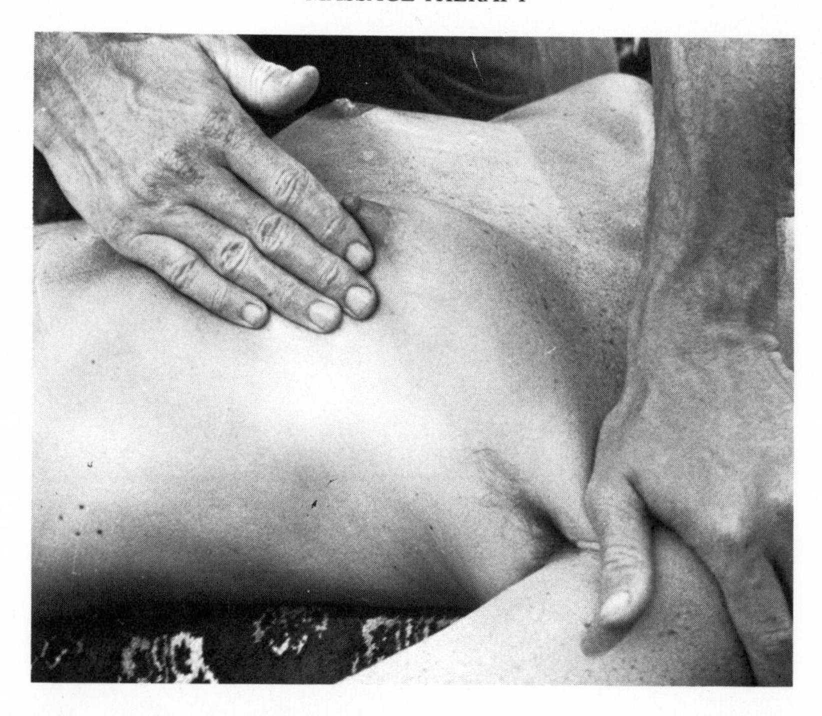

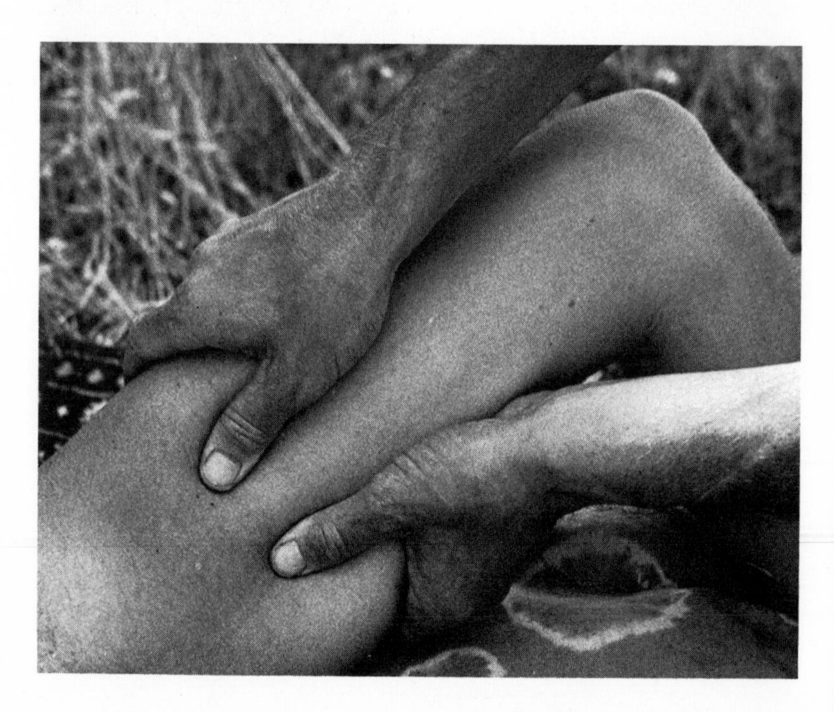

12.

Full Back Massage

The best area on which to learn massage is the full back. This is the flattest, broadest area of the body and is the area with which most massages deal. If you can learn the strokes on the back, you can easily apply this knowledge to the rest of the body.

Preparation

You will need towels, pillows, oil, and a relatively hard surface on which the receiver will lie. Do not use lotions or creams that will be absorbed into the skin. You can use coconut oil, herbal oils, scented oil, mineral oil, or even baby oil. If you ever work with someone who has a skin condition that could react to oil, you may wish to use powder.

Learn massage with someone you love and trust. Find a comfortable place where you will not be disturbed and have the receiver lie face down with a pillow underneath his stomach. This is important, because it gives support to the lower back. You may also find it helpful to prop his feet up on a pillow for additional comfort. Try not to massage on a bed. The surface is too soft and usually too low for the giver to remain comfortable. You have the option of covering the buttocks and legs with a towel for warmth and comfort. Some people are shy and may prefer to remain covered. The photographs in this book show common positions for giving a massage to obtain maximum comfort for both the giver and receiver. It is self-defeating if either giver or receiver is not comfortable throughout the duration of the massage.

It is a good practice to wash your hands thoroughly before

beginning the massage. This not only cleans and warms your hands, it also allows you an opportunity to become relaxed and focused.

I would like you to concentrate for a few moments on your hands, since they convey vitally important sensory information. Rub your hands together and feel the sensory feedback. Close your eyes and try an energy-sensing exercise with your hands. Rub them together gently, and when you feel a warmth, stop rubbing. Now, slowly move your hands a few inches apart. If you feel a warmth or energy flow develop between them, move them even farther apart and then closer together again. Make note of any change in sensation as your hands move apart and then back together. Continue this exercise for a few minutes. It may take some time for the current flow to develop or for you to recognize what is already there. Do your hands come together more easily than they move apart? Do you feel any attraction between your hands? You may experience a force field as your hands approach each other. As you become more attuned to the energies of your hands, you will be able to feel this energy flow when your hands are far apart. You may also feel a tingling in your palms, or your fingertips may "come alive." Your hands are the most important part of the massage. Take time to stimulate and develop your physical *and* energy senses. You can enhance the energy flow through deep breathing and imagery. Notice your breathing. Does your stomach bulge on inhalation? You should be breathing diaphragmatically. Review the chapter on breathing, if you need to. Remember, always try to inhale through your nose. The energies I have referred to are very subtle at first. In time, you can train yourself to become more and more aware of them. Do not be discouraged if you are not able to sense these energies right away. Senses are sharpened through repeated effort.

Procedure

If there is no one around with whom to work, continue, using your imagination.

Pour a small amount of oil into your hands and rub them together to warm the oil. Do this over a towel. By prewarming the oil in this way, you will not drip cold oil on the receiver. *Never pour oil directly on the person you are massaging.*

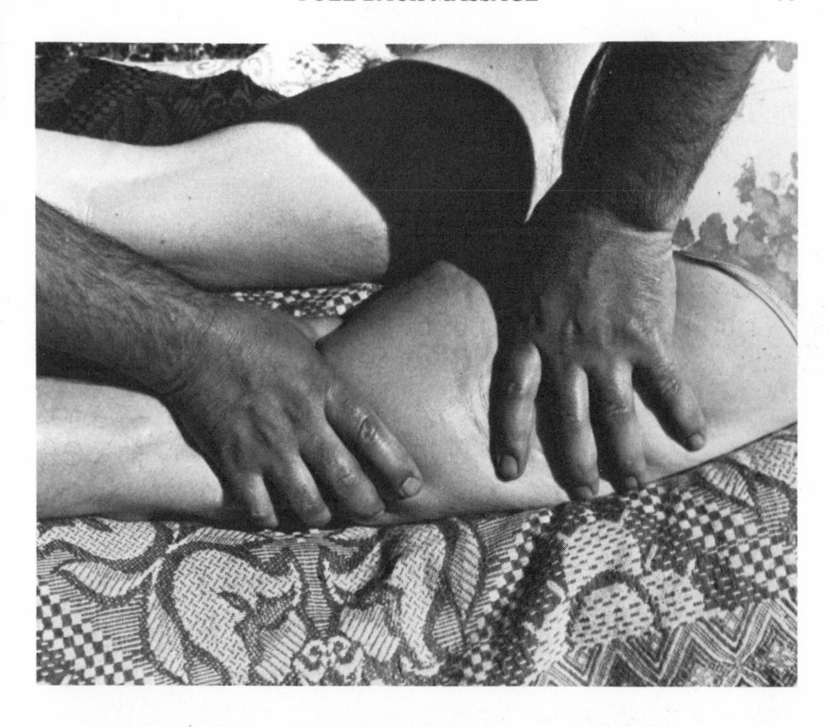

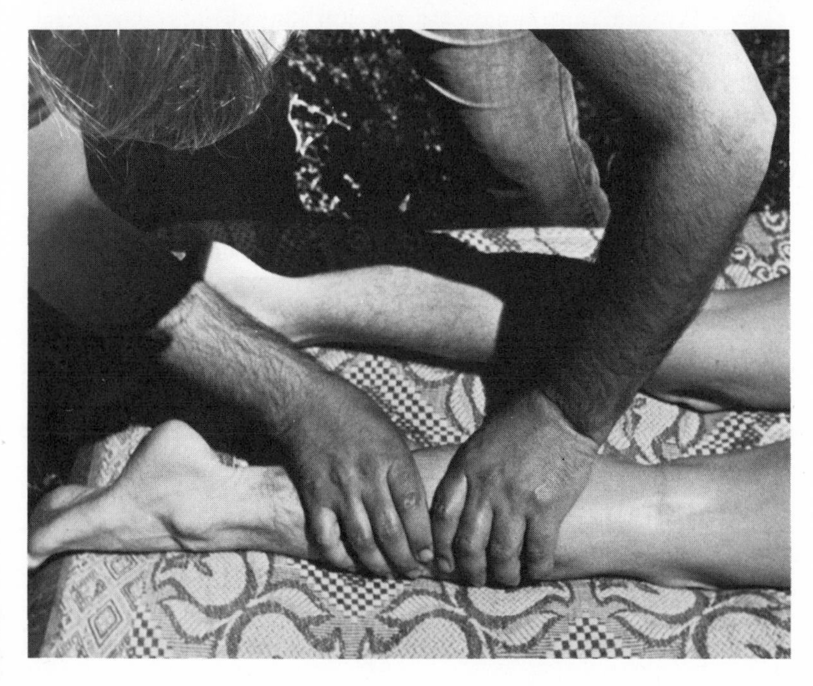

Gently spread the oil over the upper buttocks, back, and neck. Avoid over-oiling. Your hands should pass smoothly over the surface you are massaging. They should not slip and slide their way up the back. Hairy areas will need a little extra oil. Once you have begun the massage, you should avoid interruptions. If you have to reach for something, leave one hand on the receiver and reach with the other. If you are reaching for more oil, turn the hand you leave on the receiver palm up so you can pour a small amount of oil into that hand. Set the container down, carefully rub your hands together to warm the oil, and then spread it on the receiver. One further important point—*always* cap the oil. Oil is messy, and if it is spilled, it will ruin any flow and communication you have established up to that point, not to mention ruining your rug or other fabrics.

At this point you would normally do some deep-breathing and focusing exercises with the receiver. However, it will be easier for you to learn the mechanics of massage if we eliminate this part of the experience for now. When you have mastered the mechanics of massage, turn to Part 3, "The Spirit: Holistic Massage Experiences," and integrate the focusing exercises described there with your massage technique.

Next, move your hands into the starting position above each buttock. You begin with approximately twelve superficial (effleurage) strokes. The heels of your hands should be on either side of the spine as you move up the back. Never massage directly on the spine, and do not hold your hands rigidly or stiffly during a massage. Keep them loose, and let them mold to the contour of the receiver's body. As you approach the shoulder blades, let your hands flair out over the back of the shoulders. Then, reverse direction so that your hands glide over the top of the shoulders toward the neck. Move the hands up the neck and return to the starting position by drawing your hands down the spine (see Figure 11).

The first stroke is superficial, and each one following becomes progressively deeper and should always be within the tolerance limits of the receiver. You should never hurt someone during this type of massage.

During these first twelve movements, try to establish a rhythm that will remain consistent throughout the massage. Your speed of movement should be slow. The receiver will easily sense it if you hurry and may become tense with uneasiness, rather than relaxing.

Are you massaging with your arms or your body? Most people get tired while giving a massage because they stroke with their arms. Close your eyes and focus your attention on a point located about two inches below and behind your navel. This is your physical center to which I referred before. Try to move from this center. Your forward motion should be a complete body movement. This way of moving, like the diaphragmatic breath, will seem strange and even awkward at first. With practice, you may wonder how you moved in any other way.

Are you exhaling with each forward stroke? Pushing movements are best accomplished during exhalation. Review the chapter on breathing, if you have questions. Remember, return strokes are done with light pressure and should be accompanied during inhalation.

The first set of strokes is used to warm up the muscles, set the rhythm and pace of the massage, and establish communication through the hands.

As you return from your last stroke, turn so that you are facing the side of and reaching across the back of the receiver. Now start a series of petrissage manipulations. This set will take some perseverance and practice. With your hands about four inches apart, begin making clockwise motions with the left hand and counterclockwise motions with the right (see Figure 12). Continue moving from your center. These are movements that require a rhythmic rotation of your whole body.

At this point, I should enter a word of caution regarding the rib cage. The lower ribs are called floating ribs because they are attached in the back but not in the front (see Figure 9). This area can be painful if you massage too deeply. Keep pressure on the muscles next to the spine while working at the bottom of the rib cage.

Make about four circles in alternating directions in one spot and then move your hands up toward the shoulders approximately the width of one hand and continue with four more. This is a good time to concentrate on feeling the muscles and to search out pain and tightness. Use your imagination to extend your energies through your hands and into the receiver. How do the palms of your hands feel at this point?

The pressure of these circular petrissage manipulations should be almost as deep as you can make them without causing pain. Do not hesitate to ask for feedback from your partner. Eventually you

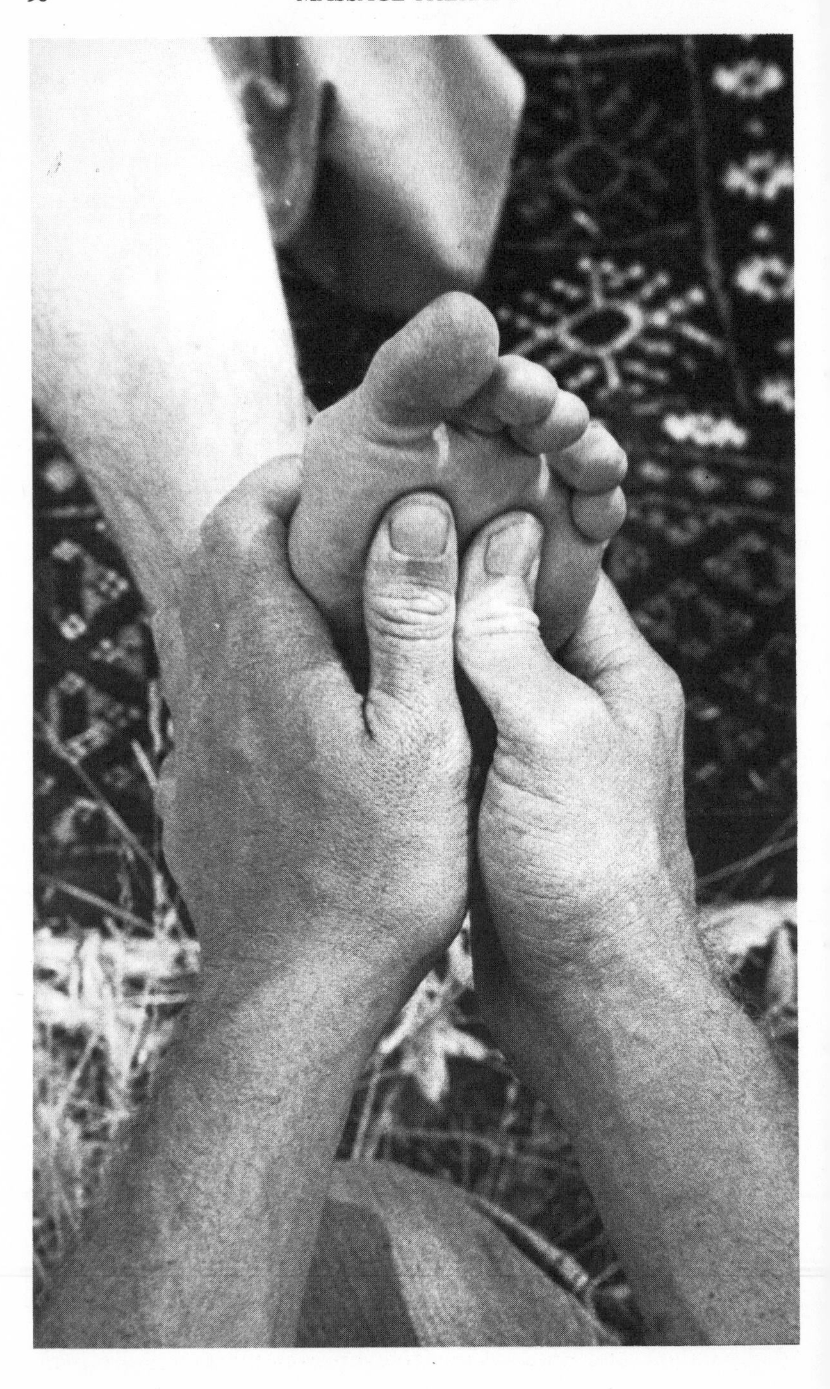

will develop a sense of touch that will tell you how deep you can go without causing pain. Commonly, beginners make the mistake of using too little pressure. I recommend that you first master the basic motions and then worry about using pressure.

Work gradually up one side of the back and then massage the shoulders with expressive circles, strokes, and kneading. It is nearly impossible to do alternating circles over the shoulders. Note the shoulder blade. It is a flat, triangular bone that slides easily over the back. Avoid pushing too hard directly on top of this bone, letting the receiver's comfort be your guide. You can certainly let your hands pass over it. Attached to the borders of the shoulder blades are muscles that very often hold tension. I like to apply deep pressure with my fingertips to these muscles, and the receiver seems to enjoy it as well. Feel free to modify these strokes according to comfort and common sense. I am trying to give you a general outline to follow. Its ultimate success depends on your own expression and creativity.

When you complete one side of the back with these circles of alternate direction, return to the starting position and do the same side again. The muscles and other tissues should feel soft. Bones are hard and generally immovable. When passing over bony areas, decrease the pressure, or you will cause pain. Remember to avoid using stiff hands. Allow your hands to conform to the body. One part of your hand may be pressing quite deeply, while another part may hardly be producing any pressure at all. Muscles in spasm are firm and painful, often feeling like hard lumps or long thin strips of very firm tissue. Again, practice improves the senses.

Following the second time you work up one side with circular motions, return to the starting position and administer the same strokes to the other side. Your fingertips should be adjacent to the spine, and the heels of your hands should be over the sides. Do the second side twice also.

How are you breathing? Are your shoulders relaxed? Remember to move slowly and rhythmically. If your arms are tired by now, I recommend that you concentrate on moving from your center.

When you have completed the two-handed circular movements, return to the opposite side, just at the top of the buttocks, and place one hand over the other (see Figure 13). This is another petrissage manipulation, and it allows you to exert even more pressure than before. Again, avoid hurting the receiver. Proceed up each side with circular motions at least once. You may do more if you prefer. Allow yourself great freedom of expression during this part of the massage. You should have a good idea by now where the problem areas lie, and you should consider giving these areas some additional attention. Muscle tightness usually settles in the shoulders and along either side of the spine. Are you beginning to gain a sense of moving from your center? When you have finished one side, repeat the procedure on the other.

Returning to the base of the spine, place your thumbs on either side of the spine and make deep circular motions approximating the diameter of a half-dollar coin (see Figure 15). Move up the spine slowly, searching for pain and tension. Avoid pressing directly on or against the spines of the vertebrae. Concentrate on the feel of the muscles in this area. When you get to the top of the back, fan the strokes out over the broad shoulder muscles. Do not forget to massage all the way up the neck. This part of the massage should be as deep as it can possibly be without causing discomfort. Some people cannot tolerate these strokes at all. If the receiver is very sensitive, you will have to use less pressure or maybe even eliminate this manipulation altogether.

After this friction manipulation, spend some time doing whatever comes naturally. Feel free. Express yourself. Try to flow with the massage experience. Use kneading and petrissage when needed.

Finish the massage with the same long effleurage strokes with which you started. This time the pressure gradient should decrease from deep to superficial. Again, focus on your hands. How do they feel? Allow yourself to experience the flow of the massage. Try to communicate with the muscles through your hands. Can you feel the receiver responding to your motions?

A full back massage should last from twenty to thirty minutes. The last stroke should be very light, and you should finish by gently wiping off the excess oil with a towel.

Here I like to end the massage with visual imagery. In Chapter 15, "The Giver," I have described the technique I normally use. It is important to reinforce the receiver's focus on his body by encouraging positive imagery and feelings. I ask the receiver to become aware of his feelings and body image. This aspect of the massage is very important. The receiver really has a chance to learn from and assimilate this experience. If holistic massage is to be effective, the receiver must make changes within himself. The atmosphere created by the massage is conducive to focusing that can begin these changes.

When you are finished focusing, leave the room and find a quiet place. Both giver and receiver should use the next few minutes to focus inwardly and absorb their experience.

Summary

I have given you the basic structure of holistic massage. The process can be summarized as follows:

1. *Preparation*
2. *Focusing*
3. *Effleurage* (superficial stroking with increasing pressure)
4. *Petrissage* (circular or deep transverse stroking)
   a. Alternate circles, twice on each side.
   b. Hand-on-hand circles, once on each side.
5. *Free expression* (kneading/petrissage)
6. *Friction* up the spine and over trouble spots.
7. *Free expression*
8. *Effleurage* (superficial strokes of decreasing pressure)
9. *Refocusing*

Throughout the massage, you should try to observe the basic components of rate, rhythm, and proper pressure gradient. Feel free to use kneading and other expressive motions in conjunction with the above strokes.

In contrast to the first nine chapters of this book, which contain numerous preparation and focusing procedures, the final three chapters describe only one focusing technique. By using just one focusing procedure, you may unnecessarily lose opportunities to expand the receiver's awareness on other levels. Thus, you can lead your receiver through some of the focusing experiences found throughout the first few chapters. Your responsibility as a giver of holistic massage is to expand the body awareness of the receiver. Applying some of these experiences to the receiver can help you accomplish this goal.

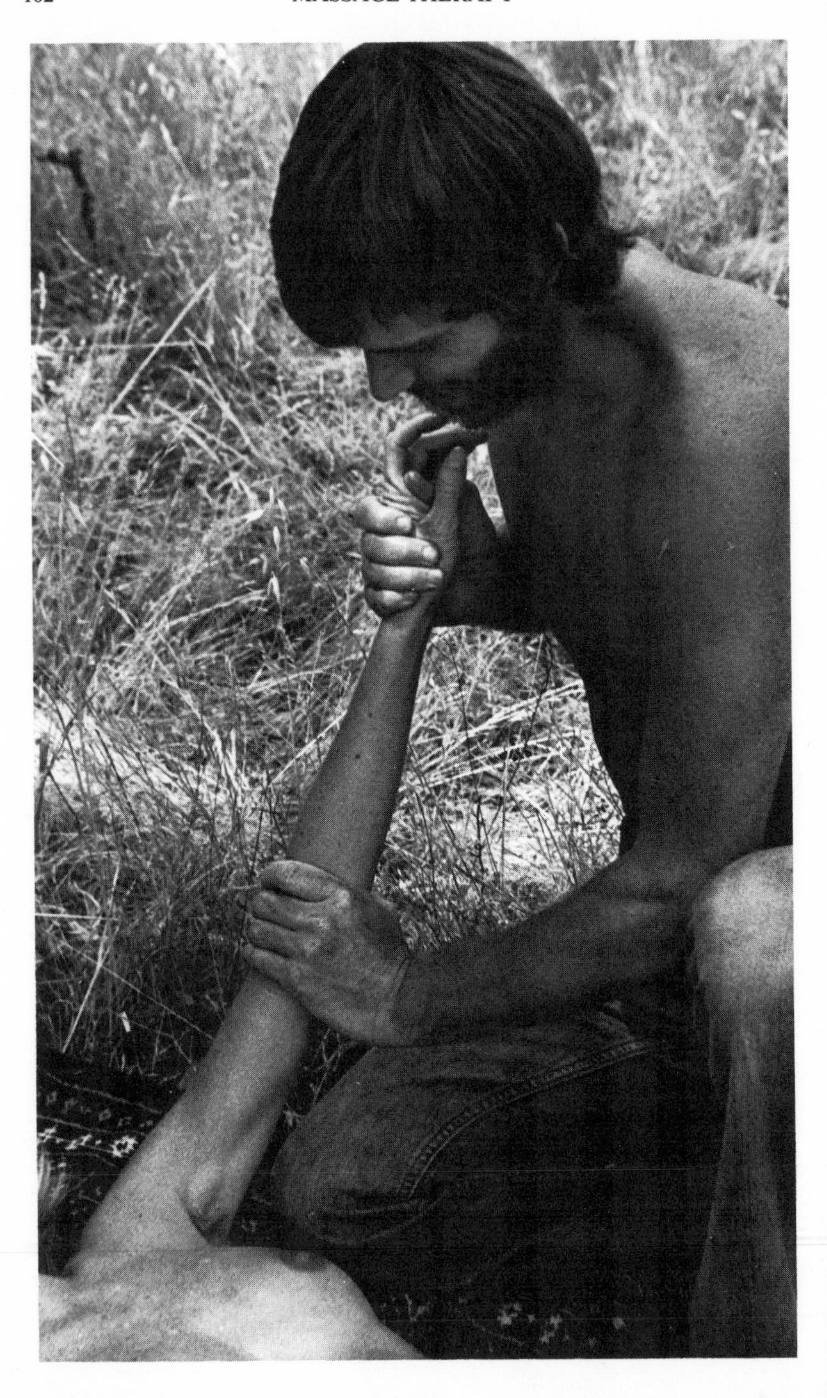

13.

Massage of the Extremities and Full Body

Extremities (Arms and Legs)

The extremities differ greatly in size and contour from the back. Massaging an arm or a leg is a more localized activity. There are large muscle masses, so friction and kneading are frequently used. There are more bony areas, so more care must be taken when massaging an extremity. These factors require the giver to have very flexible hands that easily mold to the contours of the body.

Massaging extremities also requires inventive body positioning. Get into the habit of using several pillows. Remember, massage should be as comfortable as possible for both giver and receiver. Refer to the photographs in this book for ideas on body positioning. When the receiver is on his back, it is best to put a pillow under his knees when not massaging the legs. This adds greatly to anyone's comfort.

Begin by warming the extremity with effleurage and kneading. Vary the pressure over the bones. Circular petrissage manipulations can be done by placing your hands on either side of the extremity and making circles in unison. You may find it helpful at times to support the extremity with one hand while working with the other. Follow this with expressive movements, friction, and kneading, and then finish with superficial stroking of decreasing pressure.

I prefer to massage the arms while the receiver is on his back. When working on the legs, you can have the receiver on either his stomach or his back. Experiment to see which way you prefer.

Massaging extremities is a perfect opportunity for you to experiment and allow your common sense and creativity to be expressed. I believe I have given you all the rules you need. You have to trust in your own abilities and understanding to create your own personal style and approach to massaging the full body. I know what strokes and manipulations feel good on my body, so I often use them when massaging someone else's. It is difficult to massage the extremities and full body other than the back because of the many variables. Size, shape, bony areas, and difficult positioning add up to a much more difficult massage than that tailored to the back alone. But do not let these factors stop you from developing confidence and competence in your own body massage techniques.

The hands and feet should be approached in a unique manner and should be massaged separately from the other extremities.

Hands and Feet

There are several complete volumes that describe the procedures and virtues of foot and hand massage. The underlying theory is that there are areas on the feet and hands that correspond to the various organs of the body. Stimulation of these points through massage causes a reflex energy reaction that helps balance the flow of energy to these organs (see Figure 16). This is helpful in three ways:

1. *Preventive measures:* If the feet and hands are massaged regularly, the energy meridians will be in a constant state of balance and harmony, and "dis-ease" will not easily develop.

2. *Diagnostic techniques:* An energy imbalance in an organ will manifest itself as pain in the corresponding area of the foot or hand *before* there is an observable symptom developed in the organ itself.

3. *Treatment:* When an imbalance does occur, stimulation of the proper reflex points will have a positive, curative effect on the manifested dysfunction. This is the same approach to healing used by acupuncturists in which the *energy imbalance* is treated instead of the Western approach of treating the *symptom*.

Foot and hand massage are conducted by first warming the body part. You may want to use a very small amount of oil, but it is really not necessary. Loosen the bones of the feet and the ankles.

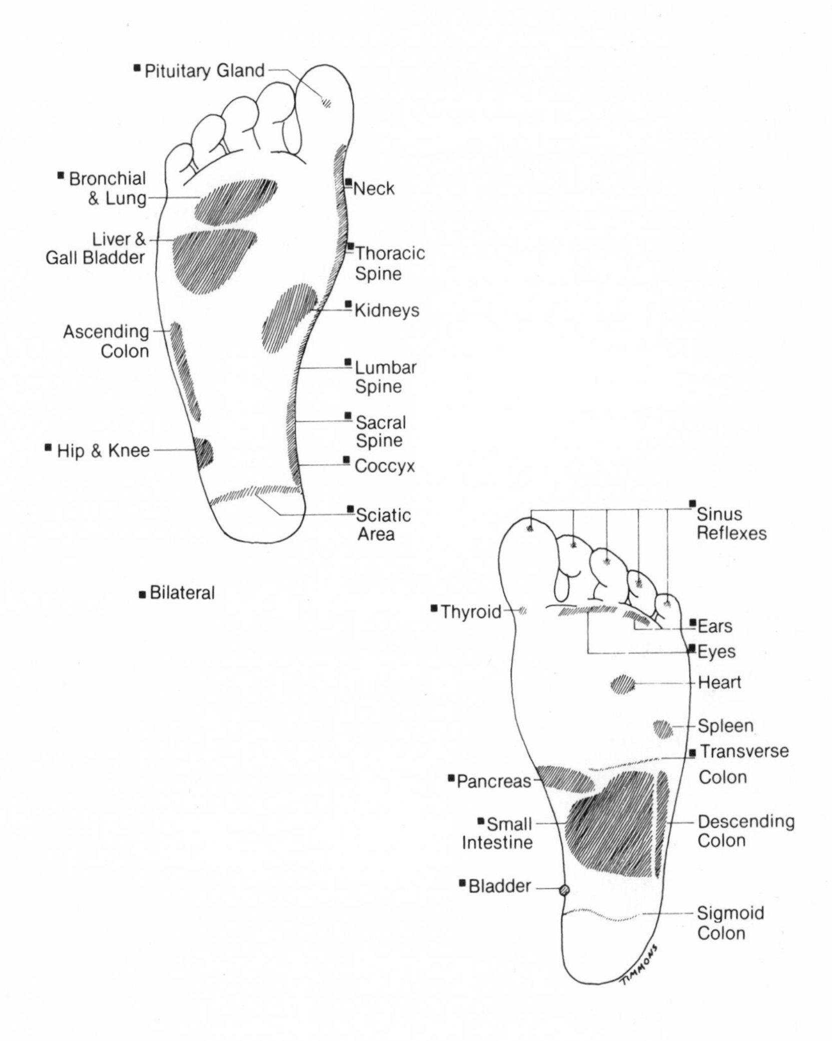

Figure 16. **Reflex Areas of the Feet.** These are only a few of the many reflex areas corresponding to bodily structures. Notice that some structures are found on either foot.

Using the broad surfaces of the thumbs, with your hands supporting the foot or hand, start at the toes or fingers and probe thoroughly, with alternating deep pressure manipulations. Press deep and then work with your thumbs in circular patterns. Always stay within the limits of pain tolerance. *Every* centimeter of the foot or hand must be covered with this same deep pressure. When you discover a painful area, pause and massage that area for a few additional seconds—again, within the tolerance of the receiver. When you have finished massaging the entire hand or foot, return to the painful areas and spend an additional short time on them. Do not try to eliminate all of the pain in one session. Foot and hand massage are not unlike that for the rest of the body. Massage is a process, not a one-time cure. Work each joint through its full range of motion, and also take a minute to squeeze the fingers or toes in succession. This will stimulate each of the five main energy meridians.

Use foot and hand massage often. You can do this type of massage almost anywhere, even with a large group of people. It is one of the most sensual of all massages. To receive a hand and foot massage feels good, and the body parts are left warm and tingling.

Get into the habit of massaging yourself. When you are relaxing, try massaging your feet. Before you know it, everyone around you will be doing the same. If a person has sensitive feet, try desensitizing them first by using the heel of your hand to stroke the soles a few times with deep pressure. Again, the most important part of foot and hand massage is your own personal expression, sensitivity, and creativity.

Chest and Abdomen

These are difficult areas to massage. The abdomen is soft, and the rib cage is hard, with a thin muscular covering. These conditions require your hands to be very flexible and your pressure distinctly variable during any one stroke.

Most women do not object to a chest massage, but they are sometimes apprehensive the first time. So if the receiver is a woman, I always ask if she would feel comfortable receiving a chest massage. The decision is hers. Remember, the purpose of massage is to promote relaxation and comfort, not to create anxiety and tension. If she agrees to a chest massage, proceed; If she does not agree, stop. Still, do not hesitate to ask the question again during the next massage. As personal contact and a level of trust develop between you, the receiver will be more open to receiving a complete, full body massage. To me, this represents a significant breakthrough for a shy, withdrawn woman, and I feel a personal responsibility to be very supportive toward this type of person.

Start with the same effleurage strokes used during a full back massage. After eight to twelve strokes, begin the deeper, circular, petrissage strokes and continue with the deeper friction. One variation I use on the stomach that you might want to try is to start just below the ribs at the twelve o'clock position. Using fingertip pressure, I make small circles at twelve o'clock, one o'clock, and so on. When I have returned to the starting position, I do the same procedure on an inner circle.

A massage of the chest and abdomen, for both men and women, is an extremely pleasurable experience. The front of the body is far more sensitive than the back. Sometimes the sides and front of the abdomen are hypersensitive and the receiver cannot tolerate massage in these areas. Again, the giver must be sensitive to the feelings of the receiver. Hypersensitivity, often the result of inner apprehensions, responds best to deep pressure and very slow movements. If the receiver gains confidence in the giver, he or she will become less sensitive. The abdomen is one of our most vulnerable spots, and it is often a major breakthrough for a person to allow another to touch this area. Be sensitive toward an apprehensive receiver. Do not try to tickle him or make any quick, unexpected moves. Such surprises will only prompt defensive withdrawal and will thus increase his tension. Your goal is his relaxation and comfort.

Face

Facial massage is a very intimate, pleasurable experience. Deep pressure is not necessary, since the muscles of the face are very thin. It is most beneficial to concentrate on expressive stroking and circles of light pressure, using the fingertips, thumbs, or heels of your hands. You need apply very little oil to the face.

The face has numerous muscles and a rich blood supply. It is another area in which concentration of tension may be found. Do not forget to do the ears and sides of the neck. Spend time with all

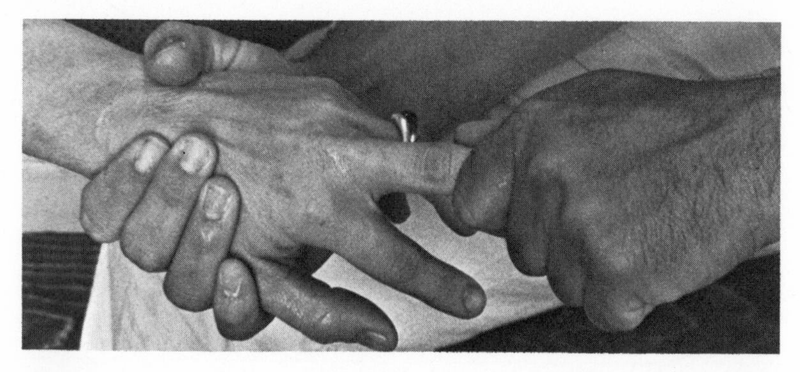

of the strokes you use on the neck. The base of the skull and sides of the neck are usually a storehouse of tension. Again, use creativity and self-expression, and finish the manipulations with long strokes of decreasing pressure. Go slowly and communicate through your hands.

Full Body Massage

The basic components of massage—rate, rhythm, pressure, and good position—are utilized during any massage. When massaging the extremities or the full body, the basic strokes and sequence remain the same as in a full back massage. The full body massage should not last more than ninety minutes. A longer experience is really fatiguing for both parties. It is good practice to have the receiver move as little as possible, so massage one side and then have him turn over. There is no special sequence in working on the different segments of the body. You should experiment to find what is right for you.

You may want to try giving a full body massage with more than one masseur. It is more fun and may be easier. The benefit to the receiver is also enhanced if he takes a hot bath before the massage, to warm and relax the body tissues. The giver's work becomes easier, and the massage is more effective.

The illustrations of anatomy included in this book will be helpful in preparing to give full body massage. But perhaps of even greater importance, use common sense and draw on your own creative resources.

Massage is an art form. And as in any artistic expression, there are basic tools and procedures. Develop your own art, and develop yourself as an artist.

PART III

THE SPIRIT: HOLISTIC MASSAGE EXPERIENCES

"I am not a teacher—
Only a fellow traveller of whom
You asked the way.
I pointed ahead—
Ahead of myself as well as you."
—George Bernard Shaw

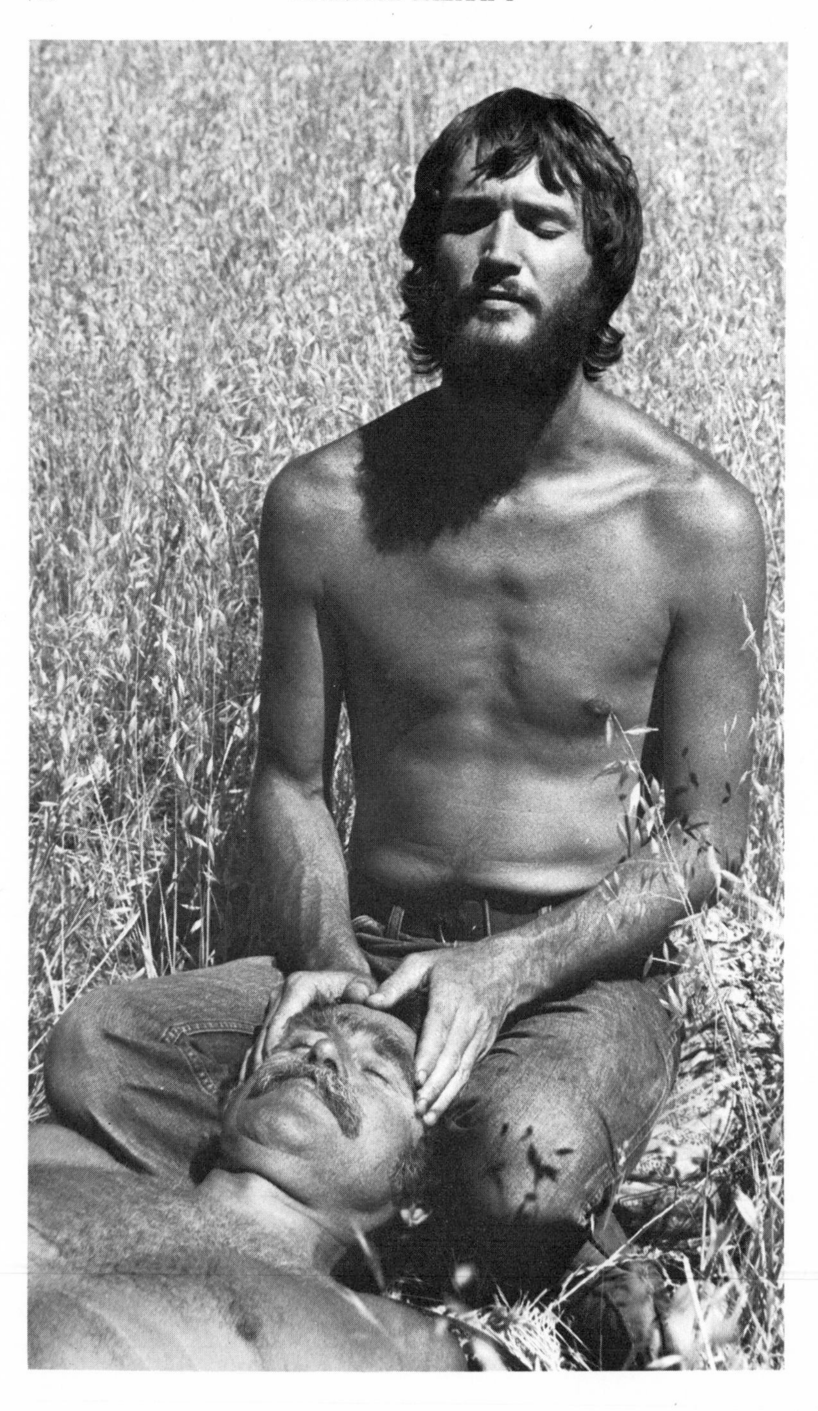

14.

Meditation/Focusing

Massage as Meditation

Massage can be experienced as a meditation. It allows the intellect to focus on an act of doing, such as the rhythmical motions of the hands and the regular rhythm of breathing. This experience can open intuitive channels to the inner healing self.

The mystical and psychic dimensions of holistic massage are most gratifying. It is an expression that is directed toward others and not just toward the self, as in other forms of meditation. This sharing of experience is very rewarding. I experience it as a joining of energies, two people working for a common purpose.

We all have a source of energy, that driving spark that gives our lives inner meaning. Some call this energy soul, or spirit, or refer to it as the subconscious, but few people deny that it exists. Most agree that the inner self is intuitive, that it knows without conscious thought. The inner self has no boundaries, so there is limitless potential for growth, experience, and creative expression. The yogis and mystics of the East say that it is possible to reach the source and become one with it through meditation. Meditation quiets the mind so that we can experience our source of being directly.

Experience

Stand up, with your feet comfortably apart and your knees slightly bent. Next, take three long, deep, diaphragmatic breaths. Your physical center is about two inches below and behind your navel. This point also corresponds to the center of gravity, or weight center, of your body. Try to get a feel for this center. You may visualize it as a point of light or feel it as a tingle or a slight movement. Breathe deeply, and with each exhalation allow yourself to relax. Try to imagine this point of light growing. Focus all of your attention and awareness on this point.

When you are completely centered, begin to move your body back and forth, shifting all of your weight onto one foot and then onto the other. Your natural tendency will be to move from your mind rather than your center. I would like you to try to imagine this motion as originating from your center. Feel the motion occurring on its own. This is what I mean when I talk about blending into the flow of a massage. The massage, or any other movement for that matter, happens on its own. We need only to blend into the perfect movement that is already happening. Moving from your center should be free-flowing and effortless.

Next, while continuing to stand with your knees bent, put one foot forward and the other back. Shift forward and back, trying to keep your back as straight as possible. Practice moving in harmony with your breath. Exhale while shifting the weight forward, inhale while shifting back. This is important, because it will help you establish body rhythm and flow during massage.

When you massage, try to feel the massage as originating from your center. With each inhalation, see the breath come in and sink deep into your center, expanding it and adding to its energy. During exhalation, visualize this energy flowing down your arms and into the person you are massaging.

If your breath and movements are rhythmical and your mind is centered, the massage will turn into a meditation. Like other forms of meditation, the results improve with practice. As you develop a feel for your natural energy flows, you will see how they can be effectively used in all physical activity.

Focusing

Techniques for focusing and centering are important for many practical reasons. They are important in helping people become aware of their natural energy and how their energies flow. Also, the giver should precede massage by leading the receiver through centering exercises in order to get both participants to focus on the same point in time and space. It is important for maximum growth and healing for both giver and receiver to be focused on the experience. While concentrating, the receiver is better able to help reduce muscle spasm and tension through conscious relaxation and imagery. The receiver is also helped to identify trouble spots on which he can work during and after the massage. I have discussed at length how massage can release stored emotional tension. This can happen only if the receiver is attentive enough to take notice of these emotions and consciously deal with them. I have also elaborated on the potential benefits of developing a sense of body awareness, and this too can happen only if the receiver is conscious of, and focused on, the experience.

Focusing is integral to holistic massage. It is one way to give responsibility to the receiver, and I believe the effects of focusing will enable permanent changes to take place within the receiver. You can use any technique you wish. The technique I describe in the section of Chapter 15 titled "A Holistic Experience" is only one possibility. As with massage, there is a basic structure to follow. But beyond this basic structure, you may either use the technique I use or make up your own. It is always good to start with a few deep, relaxing breaths and then use imagery and verbal guidance to help the receiver gather his or her awareness and energy. The final step is to have the receiver focus this attention on your hands, and you can reinforce this attention throughout the massage. With practice, you will become able to sense when the receiver is with you and when he is drifting off. When he drifts, gently pull him back by reminding him to redirect his attention to your hands.

After the massage, it is important to refocus the receiver on his body and body image. Much of the positive learning engendered by the holistic massage experience takes place after the massage. Do not overlook this important aspect of the experience.

I find massage effortless when practiced in the manner I have described. Time seems to stop, and my consciousness soars. When massage is experienced as a meditation, there is no thought of turning back. There should be only a longing to experience more.

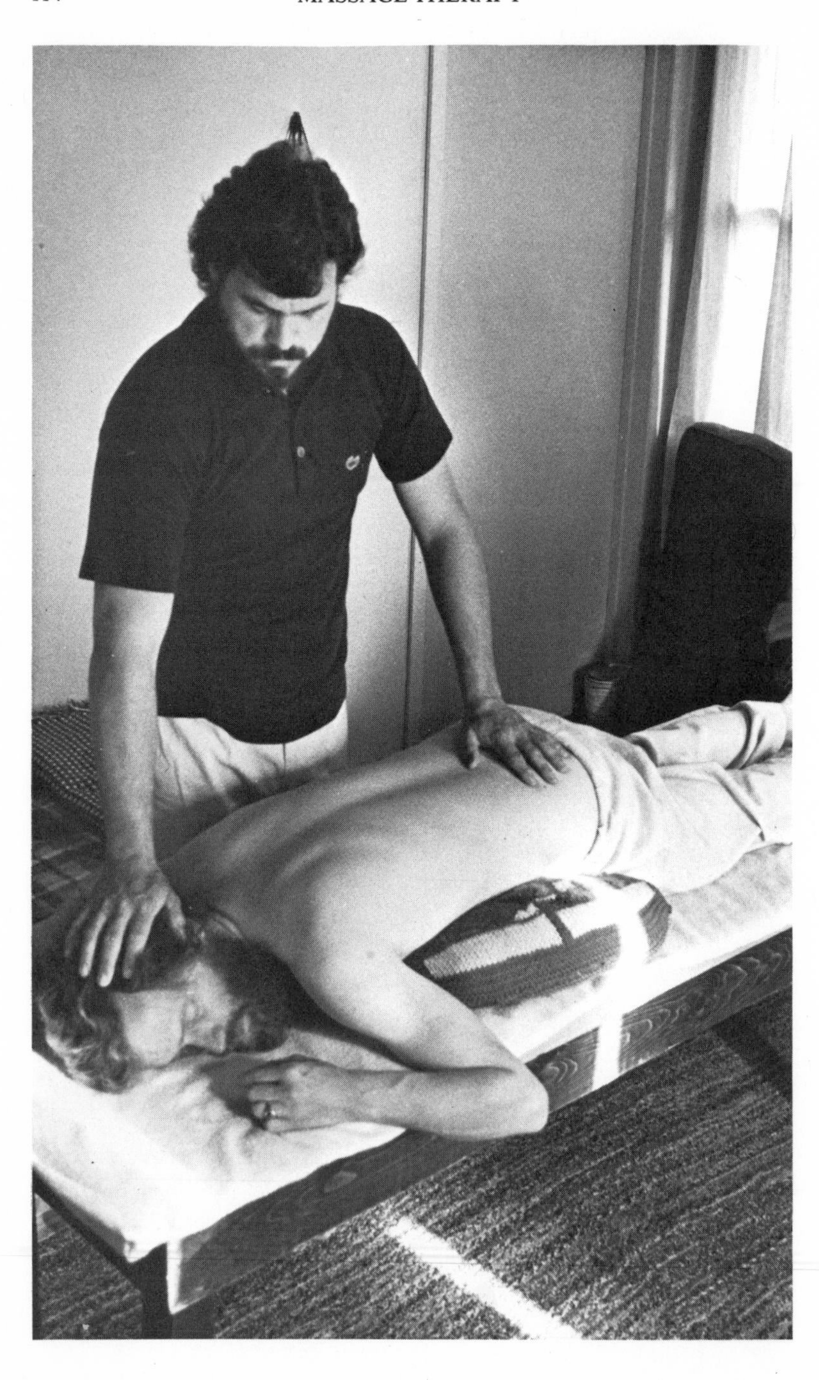

15.

The Giver

The spiritual aspects of holistic massage can be experienced by the giver during each massage session, and he may also experience inner spiritual growth over a number of holistic experiences. But what are spiritual feelings?. I am sure each of us has his own personal definition of spirituality. There will be many differences among our definitions, but there will be similarities as well. It is upon these similarities that I would like to focus for the moment.

We all have inner needs and desires. Some of these are basic physical needs, such as those for food, water, and clothing. We also have intellectual needs. The mind craves stimulation and growth. And there are still other needs that relate to the inner self. These we can classify as spiritual or psychic needs. For instance, we all need to feel that life has some purpose and meaning and that within the scheme of things our own life has some value. We seek to feel loved, needed, and wanted. Another need is for the approval and friendship of others. How many suicides are caused because the basic needs I have mentioned have not been met? There are other needs, of course. What we are basically searching for is an inner, personal fulfillment. We are searching for a harmony within ourselves, a kind of satisfaction that is not related to the material world. As these needs are met, we experience feelings of joy and contentment. It is when our basic needs are not met that we experience depression and anxiety.

Holistic massage is an excellent way to meet our basic needs, because it is a method of helping other people and a way of getting closer to them. The healing arts in general offer a tremendous opportunity for personal fulfillment. The act of helping others gives one a genuine feeling of satisfaction. These feelings are not body- or mind-oriented. They are definitely of a more personal, inner, spiritual nature. Holistic massage has the benefit of focusing the attention of the giver and the receiver on these factors. Here we are concerned with the giver.

There are personal rewards for helping a person through a physical crisis. The giver of holistic massage can often see pain turn to pleasure. It lifts his spirit to receive the gratitude and praise of the receiver. It is especially gratifying to know that the receiver not only benefits physically but learns how to help himself as well. For this the receiver is especially grateful. The basic spiritual needs of each is being met. These important inner feelings are enhanced by the focusing exercises and by a sense of shared responsibility. Holistic massage turns the attentions of both giver and receiver inward and requires them to simply feel. The results are often astonishing.

The giver who develops his art of working with the human body is often besieged with people needing help. Close personal friendships develop and grow on a basis of love and trust. The giver is valuable to both himself and others. For him, this is a never-ending source of joy. These feelings strengthen the spirit of the giver in many ways.

There are spiritual benefits for the person who practices holistic massage regularly. The very nature of the experience causes him frequently to turn his attention and concentration inward. He begins to sense feelings and energies that lie deep within himself. He gets to know himself intimately. At that point, individual differences prevent us from making generalizations. The paths the giver can travel from this point are infinite. Each person will follow his own inner instincts. These paths are definitely spiritual, because they are not of the body, and the mind is helpless in trying to explain them. Perhaps this is why we have so many disagreements when we try to define spirituality. At the point where the giver begins to explore his inner self, the guideposts stop. There are no maps or territorial boundaries. How can there be? It is an exploration into the self, and each of us is unique.

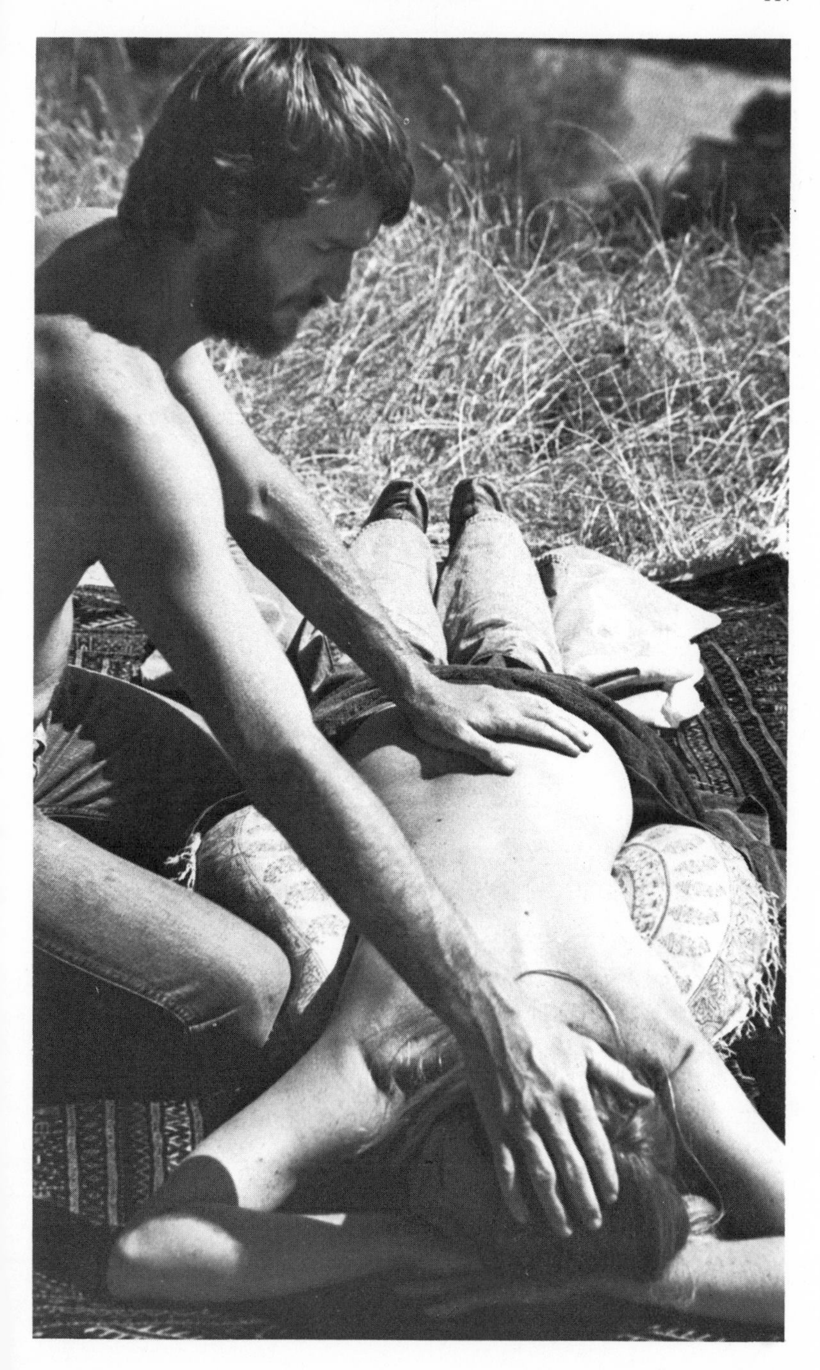

A Holistic Experience

To receive the full spiritual benefits of holistic massage, a certain structure must be followed. Giver and receiver must be focused together to experience the full benefits of the massage. It is their mutual concentration and shared purpose that separates the holistic approach from conventional massage. Let us now incorporate all aspects of this book in one representative experience. The focusing techniques are presented as a basic structure from which your own intuitions and creativity must take over.

It usually begins with a request. . .

"Oh, my back is killing me. I guess I overdid it yesterday. Dick, do you think you could do something for it to make it feel better? Maybe a massage?"

"Sure, let's go."

We seek out a warm, quiet room and ask not to be disturbed. Massage is a process that should flow from beginning to end without interruption.

I explain to my friend that during the massage we must both be comfortable. "I am going to concentrate on a full back massage, so that is the only area of your body that needs to be exposed." I point to a large terrycloth towel. "You may use this to cover the lower part of your body if you like. Please remove your clothing and lie down on your stomach. Use whatever pillows you need to get comfortable. I would like you to put one under your stomach to give support to your lower back. Get ready, and I will be right back."

I leave to wash my hands and center my attention before beginning. While washing, I breathe deeply and relax my body. I strive to become aware of the moment and let all considerations of past and future drift away.

When I return, my friend is ready. The room is dimly lit, and there is a warm, comfortable feeling in the air. I have never massaged this person before, so I have some explaining to do. "I think I should tell you that I really do not *give* massage."

My friend looks up in disbelief. "Then what are we doing here?"

"Well, you will have a massage, but one in which we both participate. In this way, you will be as responsible for the results as I am."

She looks puzzled. "How can I give myself a back massage?"

"By using the power of your imagination and conscious thought," I respond. "I do not want you to drift off. Try to maintain an awareness of what is happening and what you are feeling. The techniques you learn today can be helpful to you at other times, if your back begins to hurt and there is no one around to give you a massage.

"Now lie down, close your eyes, and take a few deep breaths." I reach for the oil and pour a small amount on my hands. I then spread the oil on her back, shoulders, and neck. When I am finished, my right hand comes to rest on her sacrum (the base of the spine), and I place my left hand on the top of her head. This maneuver uses the principles of polarity to facilitate a flow of energy along the spine.

"Take three slow, deep breaths. When you inhale, imagine your breath descending all the way into your stomach. With each exhalation, *feel* yourself relax. Allow your body to sink right into the table."

I tune my breathing to hers and begin to sense the current flowing between my hands, which are already warm. A closeness is developing between us.

"Please remain quiet during the massage. That way we can remain fully aware of the experience. I would like you to tell me if I hurt you, and let me know of any areas that are especially sensitive.

"Our bodies radiate energy. With your imagination, feel the space around your body. This is your energy space. Try to feel your energies radiating from your body. During our daily routines, we are often focused externally. Our attention is turned outward, and so are our energies. As you get a feel of your energy space, try to release all your external thoughts, as well as all thoughts of past and future. Concentrate all your attention on the present moment.

"Now, use your imagination to draw your energies and attention slowly in toward what you perceive as the center of your self. Imagine this center as a point of light or a source of feeling. As your energies and awareness converge on this point, see it grow. Focus all of your energy and attention on this one point."

As this is happening, I can feel a warmth and tingling in my hands. Breathing is slow and rhythmic.

"When you are completely focused on one point, imagine this

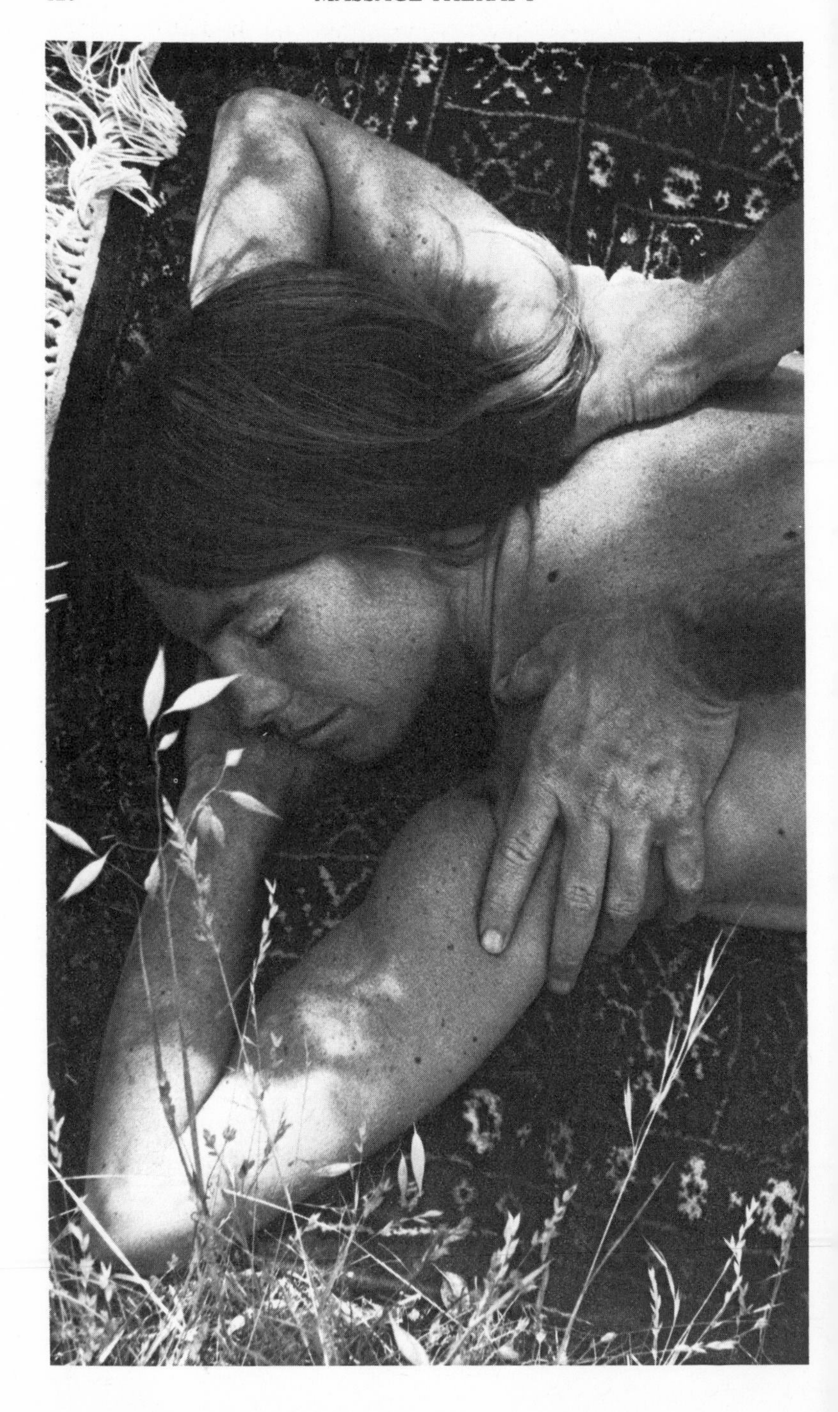

point of consciousness slowly rising within your body to a point a few inches above the crown of your head. Imagine this point of light expanding into a circle from six to ten inches across. Your awareness is completely focused on this point." I pause for a moment. "Now imagine the bottom of this circle of light open, and see the light descend into your body. Imagine the palms of your hands and the soles of your feet opening up to allow this energy to pass through your body. Feel the warmth and flow of this healing current. Notice the good feelings coming from your body.

"Energy follows thought. Wherever you focus your attention, your inner energies will follow. Allow the energy to continue flowing through your body, and move the focus of your attention to my hands."

I move my hands just to the top of either buttocks, the starting position for a back massage.

The purpose of this exercise, or focusing technique, is manyfold. First, it focuses the giver and receiver on the same thought. It also allows the receiver to concentrate and to gather all of her energy and attention on one inner point. Her concentration is further reinforced by having her move her focus of attention. With such a powerful concentration in one direction, the mind becomes free of distracting thoughts. The receiver becomes relaxed and greatly relieved of tension before the massage even begins. The visual imagery is very important. Our thoughts and feelings carry a lot of energy. You can actually *feel* love or hate directed from another. Here we are teaching the receiver techniques that she can develop to focus her energies, physical, mental, and spiritual. She directs positive feelings and energy toward herself.

"While I massage from the outside, I want you to massage with your thought energy from the inside. Your focused awareness will help you identify areas of tension, and your conscious thought and relaxation can help eliminate it. Also be aware of any subjective feelings, emotions, or images that may occur as a result of the massage. Follow your emotions, even if they are sad or unpleasant. Do not be afraid to express them during the massage. If your attention drifts, gently bring it back and focus on my hands."

Now we are relaxed, centered, and focused on the same point in time and space. I synchronize my breathing with hers and prepare to begin.

The first stroke is light and gentle. My hands move up her back, out over the shoulders, back toward the neck, up the neck, and finally I return down the spine to the starting position. As I inhale on the return stroke, I imagine energy entering my body and flowing to my physical center. All movements during massage originate from this point. It is as though the massage is happening on its own, and I am just an interested observer allowed to partake in the joys of massage without having to do any work. Massage is effortless when the mind is properly focused. The forward stroke occurs during exhalation, and I can sense the energies flowing from my center, down my arm, and into the body of my friend. I repeat this stroke approximately twelve times, gradually increasing the pressure with each stroke.

Communication, rhythm, and harmony are established during this first set of movements. I can feel her back warming, and the muscles are becoming more relaxed with each stroke. She is beginning to trust me as she becomes familiar with what is happening and what I am trying to do. I am beginning to feel a blending of our energies toward a common purpose. Feelings of joy rise within. The receiver has taken her first step.

As I progress toward the end of this first set of strokes, my mind is clear of thoughts and the massage starts happening on its own. My hands have become both a part of my friend's body, and an extension of myself.

The next set of strokes are circular and done with near-maximum pressure. This requires the rhythmic motion of my entire body. The rhythm projects my friend and me into a trancelike state. During this set, I am looking for pain and muscle spasm. My hands speak softly to the muscles and other tissues of her back, and they relax accordingly.

My head feels like I am wearing a helmet, and my ears are filled with sounds, although the room is quiet. I feel very light, and motion is effortless. There are, without doubt, many levels of consciousness. Each level has its own characteristic feelings and perceptions. From the normal waking state, one can venture through different states of consciousness and use one's changing feelings and perceptions as guideposts along the way. They mark where one has been and where one is going. And when you have traveled the roads long enough, it becomes fairly easy to find your way around.

When I get to the shoulders, I knead them and give them extra attention. Most of life's tensions seem to settle in the shoulders, and it is a rare person who has soft, pain-free shoulder muscles. Next, I spend some time working on her neck and then slowly return to the bottom of the spine to begin the same strokes again.

This time I use a little more pressure and spend some time on the problem areas I have found. As the massage progresses, my hands continue to burn and pulsate. The distinction between my hands and her back is gone. My head is becoming light now, a very pleasant sensation. The massage flows on its own with less direction and less structured pattern than before. Feelings of peace and contentment engulf me. It feels good to give a massage.

I clearly sense a blending of our energies. I can feel when my friend is with me and when she is drifting off. I know when she is in pain, and I also feel her contentment. All of this helps guide my movements and actions.

"Remember to continue to focus on my hands and massage from the inside as I work outside. Allow the muscles to relax. Feel the tension leaving your body. If you feel any emotions rising up, let them go. Much of our tension is just stored emotion, and this tension will not be released until you let your emotions go. Let down your defenses and flow with the experience."

Next, I do more circular strokes and whatever else feels appropriate. As I work on the muscles, my hands communicate love and good feelings toward them. The muscles relax and allow the healing energy to pass freely. The massage is not a struggle. It flows as effortlessly as a running river. It is easier to flow with the current than to resist it. To try to row upstream instead of blending with the natural flow would be self-defeating. The river is more powerful than I as an individual.

"Remember to focus on my hands and maintain your awareness of what is happening now. Try to breathe in harmony with me." This is easy enough to do, because now my breath is fairly loud and rhythmical.

The last set of strokes is identical to the first twelve, except that the pressure gradient gradually diminishes. I am high and exploding with good feelings. As we breathe to the same cadences the energy flow increases to a peak. There is no thought, just peace and contentment. My ears are filled with an intense buzzing sound, and my normal vision is out of focus. I have no sense of time.

When I finish the last stroke, I gently remove the oil with a towel and leave the towel covering her back. My hands come to rest again on her sacrum and the top of her head. The energy flow between my hands is very strong at this point, enough to make my friend mention the sensation later.

"Now move your focus of awareness to that point above your head and re-establish the energy flow we had at the beginning.

"Imagine the palms of your hands and the soles of your feet closing up so that the positive light energy begins to fill your body. Completely fill your arms, legs, and torso so that the light spills out the top of your head and down the outside of your body.

"When you are finished, focus within yourself and try to get a sense of your body image and of how your body feels in terms of size, shape, density, and symmetry. Sense how good your body feels. Take a few minutes to assimilate this experience, and when you are ready, you may get up and dress."

I leave the room to wash up and focus on my own experience. I feel content, high, in harmony with myself. I close my eyes and attempt to refocus in time and space. There are feelings of happiness and joy. Through holistic massage, I have had a vivid spiritual experience, and I feel as though my soul has touched another.

16.

The Receiver

by Michael Flavin

Until my encounters with the art and techniques of holistic massage, I had recurring lower back problems. After seeing several specialists whose instructions, therapy, and drug dosage regimens I followed as honestly and as closely as possible, I sought relief from a very close friend, who, coincidentally, is the author of this book. Up to this point, my only relief from pain was through conventional means that masked the pain with analgesics (pain relievers) and muscle relaxants (tranquilizers). Massage did reduce the pain to some degree at first, but not until I experienced a combined healing effect on my body, mind, and spirit did I finally enjoy lasting results.

I am writing this chapter after several complete holistic massage experiences, and the reader should be aware that a one-time, single massage is no guarantee of total well-being. Health results from a harmonious balance of the body, mind, and spirit. Holistic massage can affect this balance in positive ways, thus resulting in a healing experience, but this can only happen through repeated effort. This fact is of prime importance. Other important factors in relieving painful symptoms include confidence in the person who is giving the massage and an awareness of the fundamentals of holistic massage.

Before beginning the first in this series of massages I was to receive, Dick and I talked for an hour or so about the manifestation of pain, its relation to psychological problems, which in turn produce tension and thus intensity the pain sensations. He explained that he was not going to "give" me a series of massages, but, rather, that we were going to *share* energies of mind, body, and spirit and attempt to create a state of well-being from which we would both benefit. He said that I would be just as responsible for the results of the massage as he was.

I admit that at first I was very timid and reluctant to submit to this type of therapy, especially knowing that what my body was about to encounter was quite foreign to my own concept of physical therapy, massage techniques, and the conventional medical approach to pain therapy. Despite these alien ideas, I really wanted to try, and I opened my mind to this "new" approach, because I realized that conventional means of therapy had done little in rehabilitating my physical state. I was seeking relief from constant pain.

The first session was not immediately successful in relieving my pain, nor was the second session. I was, however, determined to follow Dick's comforting words and soothing manipulations for a few more sessions. I found that I was focusing my attention on what Dick was telling me, on what his different strokes were supposed to be achieving, and on trying to remember to breathe in unison with his movements. Focusing on these elements did not allow me to become aware of the experience in its totality. Now I realize that the first two sessions were beneficial, although my pain remained. We were laying the necessary foundation for future holistic experiences.

I am reminded of what it was like to learn how to drive a car with a standard transmission. At first, it all seemed so confusing and disjointed. With practice, however, my reflexes became more and more automatic, and I can now focus my attention on *where* the car is going, rather than *how* to get it there. In much the same way, focusing, rhythmic breathing, and cooperation necessary for successful holistic massage eventually came together.

With practice, I automatically became much better able to relax. This is one of the most important keys to a successful massage. By relaxing, you can experience a realm that was unknown to you before. As you know by now, tension causes muscle spasm, which is manifested as pain. This pain reflexively causes unconscious, increased tension, intensifying muscle spasm and pain. I understand now that holistic massage is a process. Each succeeding massage teaches me more about myself, my condition, and ways in which I can change that condition. It seems that with each session I come one step closer to total health.

As stated in earlier chapters, massage can open intuitive channels to the inner healing self. During holistic massage experiences, it is necessary to replace negative thoughts and feelings with positive ones. I have a tendency to hold on to the negative states that arise during the massage experience. I do this by experiencing these states without releasing them. I am finding that they can be released, and I am left with a feeling of relief, as if a great burden has been lifted from me. Most important, you must try to be honest with yourself. Without letting your spirit take over, the massage will not be complete. There exists an "inner self," a subconscious being that knows no boundaries and can offer us limitless potential for growth, both physically and psychologically. During the holistic massage experience, I sense that inner self as a feeling of calm, warmth, and well-being. I feel close to being whole and at peace with myself and my life.

Massage allows the healing process to begin. The experience itself does not "heal"; it merely creates the circumstances through which the healing process may begin. The spiritual awareness that results from holistic massage allows me to gain greater insights into the causes of a particular pain or area of great tension, and it is this insight that must be achieved before lasting, positive changes can take place. This heightened inner-awareness developed through holistic massage leaves me with a feeling of contentment.

In most people, this fragile awareness is shielded by years of psychological self-defense mechanisms that work reflexively. By trusting in the massage giver, this self-defense breaks down, allowing enhanced consciousness and a loss of ego. Now I find it quite common to sigh, or moan, or even cry during massage, releasing inner tension in an unconscious manner.

I look forward to entering this subliminal world when Dick and I experience a holistic massage. With the release of external thoughts, I can feel a warm flow of energy, an energy I now recognize as the real healer. This produces such good feelings within myself and between Dick and me. The heightened mind/body/spirit sensitivity allows me to identify concealed tension and allows me to release it from my body. At this point, both Dick and I experience feelings of friendship, love, peace, and harmony that overpower our senses and allows the inner sense of balance and well-being to take control.

Because with each succeeding massage my mind travels farther into this state, the effects are longer-lasting and the recurrence of severe pain is diminished. Hopefully, what has been written in these pages will afford you the same joy, peace, and contentment we have come to know.